RECOVERY FROM APHASIA

By

JOSEPH M. WEPMAN, Ph.D.

CLINICAL INSTRUCTOR IN OTOLARYNGOLOGY (SPEECH PATHOLOGY) AND
LECTURER IN PSYCHOLOGY, THE UNIVERSITY OF CHICAGO

WITH A FOREWORD BY

WENDELL JOHNSON

Director of the Speech Clinic
State University of Iowa

THE RONALD PRESS COMPANY ⋅ NEW YORK

Library of Congress Catalog Card Number: 51–687

PRINTED IN THE UNITED STATES OF AMERICA

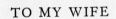

TO MY WIFE

FOREWORD

In *Recovery from Aphasia* Dr. Wepman has pointed up the crucial importance of a comprehensive approach to the problem of aphasia, coordinating the services of the speech pathologist, the clinical psychologist, and the educator, together with those of the physician and surgeon.

In this as in other fields of therapy, an evolutionary pattern is becoming fully clear: the older period of general practice was superseded by one of intense, relatively fragmented specialization, out of which is emerging an era of interprofessional teamwork that is something new under the sun. One of its most significant by-products is a new kind of specialist, who undergoes an unconventional pattern of training which includes knowledge of a variety of professional disciplines and skills that are needed in dealing with an actual speech problem.

The result is that today for the first time in history we have, in significant numbers, experts on such disorders as cerebral palsy, stuttering, and aphasia, experts who are not, in the traditional sense, neurologists or speech scientists or psychologists, but who are, in a sense so new that we lack words to express it, specialists in the therapy of a particular type of disorder. In contrast to the older general practitioner and the earlier type of specialist, we are seeing in our own day the rise of the expert who appreciates his own limitations and seeks accordingly the cooperation of other workers, from whom he learns everything possible and to whom he teaches all that he can, in the interests of the patient—not as an ear, a leg, or a tumor, but as a whole person in a complex cultural environment. That is, we are entering an age of teamwork—out of sheer necessity and none too soon. The present book typifies this new age of teamwork. Dr. Wepman insists upon placing the specific aphasic symptoms in a meaningful perspective in relationship to the patient viewed—and respected—as a whole person, in a home or hospital, a neighborhood, and a culture that must be reckoned with in dealing effectively with the patient's needs.

This is a practical treatment of professional aphasia therapy, suitable for daily use by every member of the growing team that is combating the ravages of aphasia. The team is growing partly because, as Dr. Wepman makes clear, with our modern stepped-up tempo of living the number of physical injuries in war and peace and the number of persons in late middle age who suffer cerebro-vascular impairment ("paralytic stroke") are increasing alarmingly. It is a team made up of speech pathologists, clinical psychologists, psychiatrists, neurologists, neurosurgeons, educators, nurses, and vo-cational counselors, and the work of these specialists can be greatly aided by the understanding and cooperation of neighbors, friends, and relatives. More and more frequently the team is coordinated, as it should be, by an aphasia therapist, new-style, described, and in part created, by Dr. Wepman. All members of the team need this book and will profit from studying it carefully. Its widespread use is des-tined to enrich the lives of our brain-injured, directly through more effective therapy and indirectly through the stimulation of the fur-ther scientific research that is needed. *Recovery from Aphasia* is a valuable aid for the thousands who have been awaiting the arrival of a guide of this kind.

WENDELL JOHNSON

Iowa City
October, 1950

PREFACE

This book is written for the aphasia therapist. In part it attempts to define what an aphasia therapist may be. In the author's mind, everyone concerned with the task of rehabilitating the aphasic patient falls into this category. In certain frames of reference it may be the speech pathologist, who sees his task as a re-education of the patient's speech abilities. Or it may be the clinical psychologist, whose orientation is largely psychotherapeutic and who visualizes re-establishment of the patient's personality as the greatest need. It may be the special educator, whose techniques in developing new learning are called upon to guide the recovery process. So, too, the physiotherapist, the occupational therapist, the neurologist or psychiatrist or family doctor or nurse of the over-all team of rehabilitation may each in the exercise of his or her specialty be considered an aphasia therapist. This does not complete the list, for more often than not the major burden of recovery may fall upon non-professionals—the families and even the friends of patients—whoever makes up the daily human environment with which the patient comes into contact during his recovery. These are the aphasia therapists for whom the book was written.

In any course of training that touches upon aphasia or other behavior problems following brain injury, it is believed that this book will serve a useful purpose, either as a class text or as a reading reference. Among courses which the author has had in mind in writing the book are those in speech pathology, clinical psychology, special education, nursing, occupational therapy, physical therapy, and social work.

The author hopes that the book will serve as a stimulus to broader thinking in the field of aphasia therapy, helping to remove it from the pedestrianism of daily lesson plans and word drills to the stimulating adventure in rehabilitation that it can be with a little imagination and planning.

Aphasia recovery as a field for research and therapy was originally brought to the author's attention in discussions led by Professor Robert West in his classes at the University of Wisconsin. His challenging presentation served as the original motivating force behind the years of clinical practice and research that have gone into this volume. Certain other individuals have given so much assistance in the preparation of the book that special acknowledgment of it is required. Dr. Daniel J. Sullivan and Dr. Manuel Sall cooperated during the research stages at De Witt General Hospital. During preparation of the manuscript, Dr. Douglas Buchanan in neurology, Dr. Mandel Sherman in psychiatry, and Professor Stephen Corey in education, all of the University of Chicago, edited and criticized each section from the viewpoint of their respective specialties. Dr. Joseph Reich rendered assistance by translating German texts on aphasia and making comments on the manuscript. The author's students in graduate psychology seminars in speech pathology acted as critics and advisers for a period of over two years, and another group of critics were the Mental Hygiene Clinic staff, Chicago Regional Office, Veterans Administration, especially Mrs. Sylvia Knie. The critical editing and suggestions of Professor Wendell Johnson of the University of Iowa added much in the last stages of the book's preparation. Finally, the assistance rendered by the author's wife in logical analysis of the material as it was prepared made the final production possible and meaningful. The author has made every effort to avoid errors in the preparation of the book. Any which may still remain are of course his own responsibility.

J. M. W.

Chicago
October, 1950

CONTENTS

ILLUSTRATIONS

TABLES

PART I

NATURE OF APHASIA

Chapter 1

INTRODUCTION TO APHASIA THERAPY

In the preface of his book on counseling, Carl Rogers notes a marked shift of interest among psychologists in the second quarter of the present century. He comments on the earlier preoccupation with "primarily analytical and diagnostic" material, while pointing out the more recent emphasis on "the dynamic processes through which adjustment is improved." [1] A striking parallel to the trends reflected in Rogers' statement is to be found in the area of aphasia. From the days of Broca's first description in 1870 of the role of the cortex in language production until the recent world war, the primary attention of students of aphasia was centered upon the role of the cortex in language function. Very little attention was given to the possibility of the patient's recovery. Goldstein recently commented upon the difficulty in Germany after the first World War in securing cooperation toward the "establishment of special hospitals for treatment of soldiers with brain injuries and especially with aphasic symptoms." [2] Yet nowhere else but in Germany had the idea of treatment for the disorders of language after brain injury even been conceived on such a scale. In such important studies as those by Goldstein,[3] Weisenburg and McBride,[4] and Mills,[5] which are outstanding in the early consideration of therapy for aphasia, the essential emphasis was upon diagnosis, concepts of cerebral function, and personality characteristics.

It has been only with the growth of interest in problems of adjustment in the general population that therapy for the brain-injured has gained any widespread recognition. This developing attention was greatly stimulated by the large numbers of brain-injured patients

---

[1] Carl R. Rogers, *Counseling and Psychotherapy* (Boston: Houghton Mifflin Co., 1942), p. vii.

[2] Kurt Goldstein, *Language and Language Disturbances* (New York: Grune & Stratton, Inc., 1948), p. 325.

[3] Kurt Goldstein, *Aftereffects of Brain Injuries in War* (New York: Grune & Stratton, Inc., 1942).

[4] T. Weisenburg and K. McBride, *Aphasia* (New York: The Commonwealth Fund, Division of Publications, 1935).

[5] Charles K. Mills, "Treatment of Aphasia by Training," *Journal of the American Medical Association,* XLIII (May, 1904), 1940–49.

who needed therapy as an aftermath of the second war. The medical commands of the armed services, with their awareness of the size and severity of the problem, attempted to concentrate most of the brain-injured servicemen in a few neurosurgical hospital centers. In England and in Russia, according to published reports, a similar situation existed. These groupings of aphasic patients permitted intensive study of the effects of therapy at a time when all facets of the problem of human adjustment were being subjected to earnest investigation. Experience concerning the type and degree of therapy needed for aphasic patients in one of these centers in the United States, and a comparison with the same type of experience as reported in the literature from other countries, form the basis for many of the conclusions stated in the present work.

The language disorder we are discussing is called aphasia. By definition, aphasia is any language problem resulting from organic disturbance of cortical tissue in which the defect is not due to faulty innervation of the musculature of speech, dysfunction of the peripheral sense organs, or general mental deficiency. The language problem manifests itself in the areas of symbolization, comprehension, and reproduction of concepts while the individual is using or attempting to use conventional spoken or written symbols. The brain defect which produces the aphasia is seen to produce also many other far-reaching symptoms beyond the realm of language. Many personality aberrations, many atypical modes of behavior that are not readily acceptable in our society, and various other symptoms of a functional nature are seen to be the direct or indirect result of the cerebral impairment. Recovery from the disorder of language, it is believed, is based upon over-all recovery of the individual with a new ability to function in society as a contributing part of that society. This, as is evident, is far beyond the concept of speech recovery as traditionally understood; it involves a total personality readjustment, a new-found stability as a person. It is a concept basic to the present book that recovery of the ability to speak, to read, or to write while the patient is still unable to adjust to society is a futile and useless goal. Language skill in a person unable to resume a normal or satisfying place in society is a wasted resource. A resumption of social intercourse in a manner mutually acceptable to the patient and to society, a controlled reduction of the effects of the personality aberrations which follow brain injury, stability of psyche, and insight into the physical limitations imposed by the brain insult seem to be the important goals. Language should be considered as the means of interpersonal relations, not the end result of recovery.

On the basis of this theoretical discussion of the needs of the individual, effective consideration may be given to the needs of society for establishing such a recovery and training program. At the present time there is a pressing and immediate problem which is only partially being met. During the recent war great numbers of individuals incurred injuries which produced the symptom-complex called aphasia. Some small percentage received the benefits of army training centers designed for a resolution of their problems. For the most part they were young male adults whose symptoms were the product of direct injury to the brain. Some few had suffered other types of cerebral insult such as cerebrovascular accidents or extirpation of brain tumors. It is becoming apparent through the continuing efforts of the Veterans Administration that probably an equal number sustained such cerebral disorder and consequent aphasia with all its connotations and were not given the necessary treatment before their discharge from the armed services. Some of these patients are now being reached through both in- and outpatient centers of the Veterans Administration. With the increasing numbers of brain-injured soldiers of the recent war being given routine physical examinations for pension purposes, it is becoming increasingly apparent that the wartime coverage of the psychological and language concomitants of brain injury was quite inadequate. Evidence now indicates that a much wider program is needed to accommodate all the aphasic veterans who should have psychotherapy and language training. The chances that such programs will be implemented are not as good as those directly concerned would like them to be, largely because trained therapists interested in the problem are not available in sufficient numbers. It can be said that the Veterans Administration is cognizant of the problem and in many of its installations is training new groups of therapists, or is contracting wherever possible for the services of clinics in nearby universities.

The Veterans Administration's efforts, however, deal only with the immediate phase of one part of the problem. The war made it necessary to focus attention upon great numbers of patients who needed assistance and who were concentrated in a few locations. It is unfortunately true that in the general population there are a great number of individuals, many of them elderly, who yearly succumb to cerebrovascular accidents (commonly called strokes) which leave them aphasic in some degree. The greater number of these adults have never been exposed to any form of nonmedical therapy other than the untrained ministrations of members of their immediate families. Statistics as to the number of these patients are almost completely lacking, but in many families there is either a present member or one closely related who has suffered a "stroke" and a consequent debilitation caused by cerebral damage. In one apartment hotel in Chicago the author observed five such patients on one floor. The mean age of this group was close to fifty. Each of them walked with the aid of a cane, and the limitation of movement in the right leg indicated some degree of damage in the left cerebral hemisphere. Without making a closer examination it was evident from their behavior and the behavior of their attendants that they had been accepted as suffering from a general personal and social disorder which made them continuous charges on their families. To the best of the author's knowledge not one of these individuals had ever been considered as a proper patient for aphasia therapy. Yet, from the author's experience with a sixth resident of the same floor of the same apartment hotel, the common aphasic disorder from which they were all suffering was subject to more or less successful treatment. Again without exact data, it appears that with the complexities and strains of our society there is likely to be an increasing incidence of cerebrovascular disorders. Many of the patients seen by the writer over the three years preceding publication of this book have been professional men and women in their late forties or early fifties, certainly not of an age when their contributions to society had been completed. This group of active, comparatively young people is made up of excellent therapeutic prospects. The extension of a recovery program to them appears to be a real need of our society.

With the development of increased knowledge and skill by our neurosurgeons, still another group in need of such therapy is growing in size. This includes all those patients who suffer from brain tumors and consequent operative removal of the tumorous tissue, or those operated upon for removal of focalized irritating points producing seizures, especially when the surgical intervention is within the left cerebral cortex. A prominent neurosurgeon recently confided to the author his judgment that only with the growth of a successful nonmedical therapeutic program and a consequent improvement in the prognosis for rehabilitation would the neurosurgeons extend their efforts in certain types of brain surgery to the left cortex. Operative procedures which leave the patient a life of certain invalidism, physically and psychologically, are not to be contemplated as long as the physical risks remain as high as they are in all brain surgery. With the improved prognosis for a reasonably full and satisfying life after successful surgery, however, the considered risk of operation will be more willingly accepted. For example, it is believed that many patients suffer from epileptiform convulsions resulting from focalized irritation within the left cerebral hemisphere. Many times some control over these seizures can be obtained through long and continuous medication. The patients, however, always suffer from the need for continuing the medication if the control is to remain absolute. In the past, and too frequently in the present, the neurosurgeon has hesitated about attempting neurosurgical intervention because of the danger of complete debilitation of the patient with removal of the irritating tissue in the left cortex. With any assurance that therapeusis would follow, and with increasing chances of rehabilitation, the possibility of wider favor of neurosurgical removal of the irritating tissue should follow.

Finally, the accident rates in most of our urban centers seem to be on the increase. With the speeding-up present in our more and more complex society there is the expected amount of increase in brain injury and the consequent physical and psychological concomitants. In the past these traumatic patients, too, have been considered for the most part as hopelessly injured. When aphasia has been recognized, it has usually been looked upon as an unfortunate residual of the injury and has been permitted to relegate the individual to a relatively hopeless and incompetent state.

With our increased knowledge gained through experience with brain damage during the late war, it is believed that many of these patients, in all the categories mentioned, can be rehabilitated to some degree and can lead much more useful and satisfying lives than seem now to be possible for them. This is the population, and it is not an inconsiderable one today, which in general seems to offer a significant challenge to aphasia therapists and to indicate a great need for developing what is as yet a new and complex field.

The present volume attempts to answer the following series of questions concerning aphasia and aphasia therapy: first, what is known about the disorder? second, is the disorder amenable to therapy? third, what groups should be interested in aphasia therapy? and fourth, what does the recovery process encompass?

Chapter 2

ETIOLOGY OF APHASIA

To gain a more complete understanding of the complex therapeutic task posed by the aphasic brain-injured patient, it is necessary to consider three fundamental areas of the over-all problem. First, the leading theories concerning the etiology of the disorder; second, the important nonlanguage or personality characteristics of the brain-damaged; and, third, the very extensive and confusing nomenclature that has developed in the literature. From a review of previous research the viewpoint adopted for use in the present work in each of these areas will be shown to structure the theoretical considerations developed in the later sections on therapy.

Students of cortical function have differed widely in their concepts of the etiology of aphasia. If placed upon a continuum, one end of the scale would represent an attitude of pin-point specificity of function localized in definitely circumscribed areas, while the opposite extremity would represent an attitude of complete equality of function in all parts of the cortex. Most students of these matters are to be found somewhere near the center of this continuum, believing in specialization of function but also in the over-all integration of the cortex for control of function. For ease in considering this problem, the leading theorists have been rather roughly grouped into two schools, the first believing in "localization" of function, the other holding that "nonlocalization" of function prevails within the cortex.

The "Localizationist" Viewpoint

Broca's Area.—In 1861 Paul Broca read before the Acadèmie de la Société d'Anthropologie his now famous paper on the loss of speech following pathological disturbance of the cortex. This was the first formal mention of the relation between brain disorder and language loss. The paper was entitled "Remarques Sur le siège de la faculté du langage articulé suivé d'une observation d'aphémie (perte de la parole)" and contained the following statement:

8

Aphemia, that is to say, loss of speech, results from a lesion of the frontal lobe of the brain . . . the primary site of the lesions was in the second or third frontal convolution; most probably in the latter in all cases . . . [this] puts aside for the present the idea that the linguistic faculty resides in a fixed point.[1]

Later in that year, he reported to the same group his opinion that, "La troisième circonvolution frontale parait indispensable a l'éxèrcice du langage articulé."[2] These articles fixing specific centers in the brain as being the seat of language directed the thinking and research of most neurologists for years.

Broca's articles were widely accepted and were the basis for his later belief that all the divisions of language had precise anatomical localization in the cortex. Broca's extensive research in the anatomy of the third frontal convolution of the left hemisphere and its relation to language led to the adoption of the name "Broca's area" for that zone, and the language defect that he described became known as "Broca's aphasia." While his naming of a center for articulate language is undoubtedly the contribution for which he is most noted, Broca also called attention to the importance of the left hemisphere in language faculties and in his writings differentiated between the clinical signs in "aphemics" and "amnesics." Broca's work largely centered on the expressive language problems, with abolition of articulated language while the ability to articulate remained.[3]

Bastian's Work on Localization.—Bastian, in 1869, defined additional areas for localizing auditory and visual word centers, and centers for the tongue and hand. He was also one of the first to use diagrams to illustrate his theories.[4]

By the use of his diagrams Bastian showed the exact location of a particular lesion which was necessary to produce the language behavior observed. The diagrams were also used to show how the various parts of the brain interacted to produce language. He be-

---

[1] Paul Broca, "Rémarques Sur le siège de la faculté du langage articulé suivé d'une observation d'aphémie," *Bulletin Socière Anatomique de Paris,* XXXVI, 2ᵐᵉ série (August, 1861), 331. "L'Aphémie, c'est a dire la perte de la parole . . . a étè la conséquence d'une lésion de l'un lobe antérieurs du cerveau . . . le siège primitif de la lésions était dans la séconde ou dans la troisième circonvolution frontale; plus probablement dans cette dernière en tous cas . . . écarter aujourd'hui l'idèe que la faculté du langage articulé réside dans un point fixe."

[2] Paul Broca, "Nouvelle Observations d'aphémie produite par une lésion de la troisième circonvolution frontale," *Bulletin Société Anatomique de Paris,* XXXVI, 2ᵐᵉ série (November, 1861), 393.

[3] *Ibid.,* p. 389.

[4] H. D. Bastian, *The Brain as an Organ of the Mind* (London: Kegan Paul, Trench, Trubner & Co., 1880), p. 68.

lieved that all language problems could be divided into two groups, those involving comprehension difficulty in which the physical defect was located in the "sensory" centers or the connections between the "sensory centers and the higher centers," and those involving speaking difficulty without defect in comprehension. Bastian believed there was anatomical defect in the connective neural tissue between the "cortical gray matter and the center for muscular control of the movements of speech." [5]

Wernicke and the Sensory Centers.—Not long after this English contribution to the structural viewpoint, the German neurologists began to add the results of their research. Most noted of the German scientists was Wernicke. In his first published study he added the concept of the "sensory centers" or the receiving zones of the brain. Writing in 1873, he described an auditory center in the first temporal convolution.[6] From this concept of an aphasia due to difficulty in the receiving mechanism of the cortex, as distinguished from the aphasia described by Broca in the motor cortex, originated the dual viewpoint of brain function. Wernicke agreed with Broca that the frontal convolution was properly the center for articulated language, but held that the temporal convolution was the site for the reception of auditory impulses on the level of comprehension. Wernicke's work was so widely accepted that the temporal convolution he described was called "Wernicke's area," and the aphasia "Wernicke's aphasia."

Wernicke also defined an aphasia caused by a defect in the conducting mechanism between the temporal center and the cortical areas, as well as a total aphasia in which both the auditory reception center and the motor center, described by Broca, were destroyed.[7] Lichtheim, using Wernicke's data, produced a diagram to show more exactly how defects affected the function of the brain.[8] These diagrams were used by all the structuralists of that time.

Charcot: The Writing Center.—Charcot developed the idea of the writing center. He agreed with Broca's definition that the third prefrontal convolution was the seat of spoken language but limited his conception of aphasia to the motor type, saying: "Les lésions qui consent l'aphasie siègent habituellement dans le point indiqué par

---

[5] *Ibid.*, p. 110.
[6] C. Wernicke, cited in T. Weisenburg and K. McBride, *Aphasia* (New York: The Commonwealth Fund, Division of Publications, 1935), p. 10.
[7] *Ibid.*, p. 12.
[8] L. Lichtheim, cited in E. Froeschels, *Speech Therapy* (Boston: Expression Co., 1933), p. 48.

Broca." [9] Charcot's belief that there was a difference between a "motor" and a "sensory" defect on the highest cortical level was a major point of disagreement among neurologists of that day. In his diagram he placed a center for "ideation," which he believed served as an integrating force for all the other "centered" cortical activity.[10] He also for the first time observed the differences in behavior which could exist between individuals suffering from the same or similar neurological defects. From this he postulated the existence of different kinds of individuals. Some he said were visual-minded and some auditory-minded. Thus, a defect in the visual center in a visual-minded person caused greater failure than a defect in a visual center in an auditory-minded person.[11]

At about the turn of the century Charles Mills contributed a whole series of papers on "The Cerebral Zones of Speech." A precise structuralist, he believed that there was "extreme differentiation of the brain into functional areas, subareas, and centers." He differentiated a motor center, an auditory speech center, a visual center, and a graphic center. He led a verbal attack on the viewpoint held by Marie, defending the Broca concept that there existed for language purposes within the brain separate "motor, auditory, and visual imagery centers." [12] Although granting that the intellectual component in aphasia had received too little attention, he stated that it was due to the "sensorial disturbances and the destruction of sensorial cerebral centers and of the structures connecting these centers with other parts of the brain." [13] Mills was one of the first to view the practical aspects of aphasia, its medicolegal considerations, and, more particularly for our purposes, the treatment of aphasia by training.

Modern Structural Concepts.—In more modern times, too, the localization school has had its supporters. While these are not as numerous as they were in earlier days, what they lack in numbers is more than balanced by the vigor of their assertions. Most prolific of this group is Henschen. Denying the value of any other view, Henschen reviewed over 1,500 cases that appeared in the literature and sixty of his own cases to support his structural theory. He care-

[9] J. M. Charcot and A. Pitres, *Centres moteurs corticaux chez l'homme* (Paris: Reuff et Cie, 1883), p. 27.

[10] J. M. Charcot, cited in Henri Pieron, *Thought and Brain* (London: Kegan Paul, Trench, Trubner & Co., 1927), p. 151.

[11] J. M. Charcot and A. Pitres, *Étude Critique et Clinique de la localization matrices* (Paris: F. Alcan, 1883), p. 218.

[12] Charles Mills, "Aphasia and the Cerebral Zones of Speech," *American Journal of Medical Science,* XVI (March, 1904), 375–77.

[13] Charles Mills, "The Naming Center," *Journal of Nervous and Mental Diseases,* XXI (January, 1895), 1011.

fully tabulated the anatomical findings and believed that in every case he could identify the language defect from the area affected by the lesion. His text is a most unusual collection and is a valuable source of pathological reports. He added to the centers already named a center for music and one for arithmetic. He postulated thirty different specific locations within the brain that subserved particular functions. He recognized the delimitation of Broca's area for motor speech, discarding as unproved the work of others who wished to extend the area.[14]

The structural approach to mental activities has also found support in Nielsen's recent book on aphasia. He said, "When deciding to approach the problem from the standpoint of cerebral localization, it was not with the idea of ignoring psychology, but while taking it into full account, to stress anatomy and physiology." [15] This book is well annotated; exact cerebral defects are described and pictured in it, and the relation between observed language problems and particular organic defects is clearly made.

In a series of unpublished manuscripts,[16] the noted Russian psychologist Alexander Luria discussed a new topographical consideration of aphasia. Luria offered two completely structural concepts. First, the theory that recovery from aphasic language disorders depends on "incomplete dominance." Thus a subject with a completely dominant left lobe who had an extensive destruction of this lobe would not be able to recover language ability, while an incompletely dominant individual would. In the latter group, incomplete dominance indicates that the right lobe is already prepared to take over the task of the destroyed area in the dominant lobe. This theory is not substantiated by objective data. The whole style of Luria's writing is discursive rather than objective.

In his second theory, Luria states that one can divide the cortex into "basic speech zones" and "intermediate speech zones." The former, he believes, are the junction points of many stimuli and subserve the total act of speech. The latter are association areas which subserve only specific parts of speech. Thus a destruction of one of the basic zones results in a complete and far-reaching aphasia, while

---

[14] S. E. Henschen, cited in Weisenburg and McBride, *Aphasia*, pp. 29–30.

[15] J. M. Nielsen, *Agnosia, Apraxia, Aphasia* (New York: Paul B. Hoeber, Inc., Medical Book Department of Harper & Bros., 1946), p. 28.

[16] Alexander Luria, "Essay on the Theory of Traumatic Aphasias," unpublished MS. loaned by Jacob Heiman, editor, *The American Review of Soviet Medicine,* New York; "Factors Evoking Spontaneous Recovery of Language Functions after Traumatic Aphasia," unpublished MS. loaned by Helen Black, literary agent of the U.S.S.R., New York; "Topical Syndrome of Traumatic Aphasias," unpublished MS. loaned by Helen Black, literary agent of the U.S.S.R., New York.

absence of function of an intermediate zone could affect only the particular part of language served by that zone. This theory, too, is worthy of consideration. In terms of localization it is not unlike the theory held by many nonlocalizationists who recognize that injury to certain areas does produce aphasia, even though they believe it is a function of the whole brain to produce language. Luria's insistence upon such wide areas for his basic zones, however, as well as his attempt to fix an exact relationship between the site of the physical defect and the type of language defect, places him closest to the position held by the structuralists.

No attempt has been made here to cover all the literature on the subject of cerebral localization of function. The studies discussed are, however, considered to be outstanding contributions in the field.

The "Nonlocalizationist" Attitude

The Work of Hughlings Jackson.—Many neurologists and psychologists interested in aphasia go back to the writing of Hughlings Jackson for their first principles and most lasting theories. While he was working in England, at the same time that Broca worked in France, his analysis of and insight into the problems of language and the functions of the brain remained relatively unknown; they were rediscovered in the early years of this century. Jackson formulated, long before our present schools of psychology, a concept of the dynamic behavior of the individual.[17] He believed that the defect involved in posttraumatic language problems concerned the individual's ability to "propositionalize." He defined this term as being a relation among words that brings a new meaning not by the mere addition of the separate meanings of the words used, but rather their modifications, one upon the other. "Single words," said Jackson, "are meaningless and so is any unrelated succession of words. The unit of speech is not the word but the proposition formed by the interaction of all the words used."[18] He wrote that in aphasia there is a loss not only of the ability to propositionalize aloud but also of the ability to do so internally. He introduced the most basic of concepts, that *"the evolution and dissolution of the nervous system shows a hierarchy of functional levels, with successively higher levels developing later and breaking down sooner in the process of dissolution."*[19] He observed that many of his aphasic pa-

---

[17] Hughlings Jackson, cited in "Hughlings Jackson on Aphasia," edited by Henry Head, *Brain*, XXXVIII (October, 1915), 8–10.
[18] *Ibid.*, p. 10.
[19] *Ibid.*, p. 12.

tients could use what he called automatic speech even though they were totally incapable of expressing a proposition. This automatic speech he believed was expressive of feeling tone and attitude, even though it was not on the high level of symbolic utterance. On this he commented, "With propositional speech breaking down at the highest level, it made automatic speech that much easier on the lower level." [20]

Recognizing the impact of the work of Broca and the developing localizationist viewpoint being expressed more and more by the neurologists of the day, Jackson said, "Whilst I believe that the hinder part of the third frontal convolution (Broca's area) is the part most often damaged, I do not localize speech in any such small area of the brain." [21] He was aware of the danger of the trend of claiming exact localizing centers, for in his lectures in 1864, just three years after Broca's historic paper, he warned that "it is well to insist again that speech and words are psychical terms; words have of course anatomical substrata or bases as all other psychical states have, but we must not say that the 'memory of words' is a function of any part of the nervous system, for function is a physiological term." [22] He then promulgated what has since become one of his most quoted principles, "To locate the damage which destroys speech and to locate speech are two different things." [23]

Jackson was the first to realize the importance of a psychological approach to an understanding of the problems of the aphasic patient. Many of the principles which he first developed are, the present writer believes, still fundamental to an understanding of the dynamics of the behavior of these patients. These Jacksonian principles include:

1. No narrowly defined area in the cortex as the center for language
2. Usefulness of the clinical-psychological approach where observation of the patient takes precedence over study of autopsy material
3. Concept of higher and lower levels of behavior, wherein the loss of voluntary behavior frees the involuntary act
4. Theory of the dissolution of behavior in individuals with aphasia
5. Recognition of the nonlanguage factors which are disturbed in aphasia
6. Appreciation of the close relationship between thought and language, and his observation that they were not one and the same thing

---

[20] Hughlings Jackson, cited in Weisenburg and McBride, *Aphasia*, p. 11.
[21] *Ibid.*, p. 18.
[22] *Ibid.*, p. 13.
[23] Jackson, cited in *Brain*, XXXVIII (October, 1915), p. 27.

Jackson's Followers.—While Jackson's work went comparatively unnoticed as the majority of neurologists clung to the concept of exact anatomical localization rather than the more complex and subjective clinical analysis, his work was followed closely by his students in England. One of these, Gowers, demonstrated to his students in 1900, in his still celebrated lectures on "Diseases of the Brain," the importance of considering the activity of the total cerebral cortex in language and in thought.[24]

In 1906 Pierre Marie's paper on cortical function and localization caused considerable discussion. He held that the idea of establishing separate centers was erroneous and that it was unreasonable to think that the impulses conveying the elements of speech were fixed in different localities. To Marie, speech was an intellectual function for the adequate performance of which a particular portion of the brain was set aside, and consequently damage to this portion would produce more or less failure in speech as a whole rather than any particular element of it. The degree of defect, he believed, would vary according to the intensity of the lesion and the education of the individual.[25] Marie studied the cases Broca reported and pointed out anatomical considerations that he believed indicated an error in that neurologist's conclusions.[26] In a later context he indicated that every case of aphasia that he had examined had difficulty in reading, writing, spelling, and arithmetic. Pantomime, he believed, was frequently affected, as was grammar.[27] This was probably the first recognition that aphasia was not limited in its language deficit to the area of speech but extended into every part of the communication act.

Early in the twentieth century Arnold Pick, in Czechoslovakia, was so impressed by his reading of Jackson's work that he dedicated his own classical study on aphasia to his English predecessor. Pick believed, as did Jackson, in the necessity of total cortical integration for the production of language.[28] Shortly after Pick's work was published on the Continent, Henry Head, an English neurologist, wrote a widely quoted analysis of modern studies of aphasia. This two-volume book of over a thousand pages reviewed at great length the contributions of Hughlings Jackson and served to re-

---

[24] W. R. Gowers, *Diseases of the Brain* (London: J. & A. Churchill, Ltd., 1885), p. 120.

[25] Pierre Marie, cited in H. C. Thompson, *Diseases of the Nervous System* (New York: Funk and Wagnalls Co., 1915), p. 96.

[26] Pierre Marie, cited in F. Moutier, *L'Aphasie de Broca* (Paris: G. Steinheil, 1908), p. 104.

[27] Pierre Marie, "Étude Clinique sur les modalités des dissociations dans les lésions encephaliques," *Revue Neurologique*, XXIX (1922), 14.

[28] Arnold Pick, cited in Weisenburg and McBride, *Aphasia,* p. 11.

establish a "Jacksonian school," a psychological approach to aphasia. Head, however, did much more than review Jackson's work; he gave direction to the psychological approach, analyzed the concepts, and produced a viewpoint which is widely accepted today. Head said, "I have combined under the general heading of symbolic formulation and expression the disorders of language produced by a unilateral lesion of the brain, because in the majority of instances the gravest disturbance is shown in the use of such symbols as words and figures." "In Aphasia," he went on, "any act of mental expression which demands symbolic formulation tends to be defective, and the higher the propositional level the greater difficulty will it present." [29] This appears to be a restatement of the Jacksonian position with the added concept of abstraction, for Head recognized that the acts of greater symbolic formulation were the more complex acts which required a greater degree of abstraction in their fulfilment. Head mentioned some of the very few cases appearing anywhere in the literature of individuals who had recovered language through training . . ." [30]

Views of Modern Neurologists.—Many modern neurologists follow the basic precepts of the "non-localizationist" viewpoint. In his excellent treatise *Brain and Mind,* Berry said, "There is probably no word, still less a collection of words, expressing an idea which does not involve the activity of practically all parts of the cerebral cortex, and it consequently follows that diagrams purporting to represent the speech center as being solely in Broca's area should disappear from the textbooks." [31] Berry said later that "speech results from a multiplicity of neurons interrelated through the cerebral cortex with specialized functional areas at certain points." [32]

No more signal contribution to the recent history of aphasia has been made than the work of Kurt Goldstein. Since a considerable portion of his attention was centered upon the re-education processes, much more will be said of his studies in other sections of this paper. Goldstein worked in Germany after World War I with soldiers who had cerebral injuries. He concluded that one could grasp the total problem of the aphasic adult only by the concepts of Gestalt psychology. [33] His attitude toward localization is best understood in that

---

[29] Henry Head, *Aphasia and Kindred Disorders of Speech,* 2 vols. (New York: The Macmillan Co., 1926), Vol. I, p. 212.
[30] *Ibid.,* Vol. I, p. 364.
[31] J. A. Berry, *Brain and Mind* (New York: The Macmillan Co., 1928), p. 409.
[32] *Ibid.,* p. 411.
[33] K. Goldstein, *Aftereffects of Brain Injuries in War* (New York: Grune & Stratton, Inc., 1942), p. 64.

frame of reference. He said, "To every mental performance there corresponds a dynamic process which concerns the entire cortex. The function of a specific region is characterized by the influence which the particular structure of that region exerts on the total process." [34] In another context, Goldstein was even more explicit when he said, "Localization of a performance means to me not an excitation in a certain place but a dynamic process which occurs in the entire nervous system, even in the whole organism, and which has a definite configuration for each performance . . . a specific location is characterized by the influence which a particular structure of that area exerts upon the total process, i.e., by the contribution which the excitation of that area, by virtue of its structure, makes to the total process." [35]

Goldstein formulated a series of laws of the disintegration of function. These have made re-education a more rigorous discipline than it was before. They include:

1. A single performance or performances in a specific field (e.g., visual, motor) will never drop out alone. Invariably all performance fields are affected, although the degree varies to which the individual field is envolved.

2. A single performance field will never drop out completely. Some individual performances are always preserved. [36]

Working in the same area, Halstead, at the University of Chicago, has been able to demonstrate that the individual after brain injury shows an inability to categorize, to shift, and to group things conceptually. [37] Probably no one working in the field of picturing the activity of the cerebral cortex has done more to clarify the activity of the frontal lobe than Halstead. Working with his own carefully constructed battery of tests, he has been able to measure the function of this lobe, which previously has been considered one of the more silent areas of the brain. In one of his early papers on frontal lobe function, Halstead indicated that while a basic substratum of cortical tissue may affect and be related to a particular function, damage to one section may affect another, since "both parts may have formed a unit and the inactivity of one due to its damage has set out of function the whole apparatus. Consequently, we must distinguish between indirect effects and secondary effects; the first produced by an

[34] *Ibid.*, p. 82.
[35] *Ibid.*, p. 84.
[36] K. Goldstein, *The Organism* (New York: American Book Co., 1939), p. 28.
[37] Ward C. Halstead, "Behavioral Effects of Lesions of the Frontal Lobe in Man," *Archives of Neurology and Psychiatry,* XL (October, 1939), 783.

influence of abnormal events in one part of the nervous system upon another part, while the second are the sequelae of isolation." [38]

The studies of Lashley, now of Harvard University, have stirred more controversy than any similar reports since Marie's denial of the classical location theories early in the century. Lashley removed increasing amounts of cortical tissue from the brains of rats and observed their learning behavior. His observations led him to postulate that "the whole implication of the data is that the 'higher level' integrations are not dependent upon localized structural differentiations, but are a function of some more general, dynamic organization of the entire cerebral system." [39] This generalized ability of the cortex he explained by his theory of equipotentiality of cortical matter. In another context he explained the basis of localization as apparently the grouping of cells of similar function within more or less isolated nuclear fields,[40] but he argued that his data showed that "in addition to their specific functions all parts of the cortex exercise a general facilitative effect upon the rest." [41]

These are the major proponents of the nonlocalizationist viewpoint. In number the studies reported represent only a small proportion of the research that has led to the opinion that the brain functions as a whole. Most of the work reported has been selected because of its importance in the total picture of the nonlocalization school.

Viewpoint of the Present Book

Research by other students of aphasia has led the writer to accept as a rationale for the approach to re-education discussed here the following working principle : *Aphasic language disorders are considered as affecting all the language modalities and cannot be limited to specific language skills. The recovery process must include a program leading to reintegration of the activity of the cortex and not to specific skills. While not overlooking the contribution of the "localizationists," the writer believes that a more hopeful prognosis can be made for aphasic adults with the acceptance of a nonlocalizationist viewpoint in accordance with which recovery follows reintegration of the remaining cortical tissue into a functioning whole.*

[38] Ward C. Halstead, "Preliminary Analysis of Grouping Behavior in Patients with Cerebral Injury," *Journal of Psychology,* XX (May, 1940), 13.

[39] K. S. Lashley, "Factors Limiting Recovery After Central Nervous System Lesions," *Journal of Nervous and Mental Diseases,* LXXXVIII (October, 1938), 741.

[40] K. S. Lashley, "Functional Determinants of Cerebral Localization," *Archives of Neurology and Psychiatry,* XXXVIII (August, 1937), 371.

[41] *Ibid.,* p. 385.

Chapter 3

NONLANGUAGE CHARACTERISTICS OF APHASICS

It has been pointed out that the major interest in intracranial pathology in the past centered on the complexities of cortical function. During the period between the two world wars, however, there developed a growing mindfulness of the possibility of recovery from some of the debilitating effects of brain damage. Especially after 1930, speech pathologists concerned themselves with therapeusis directed at the most evident of the aphasic disturbances, the reception or production of speech. Almost simultaneously, psychologists and psychiatrists were increasing their interest in dynamic diagnostic procedures and resolution of adjustmental problems in the general population. In the course of their studies they collected a considerable body of data concerning the abnormal behavioral manifestations found in patients after cortical disruption. Added to these data were the clinical observations of many neurologists, neurosurgeons, and neuropsychologists made on brain-injured patients. A considerable number of findings of common or expected nonlanguage phenomena seen subsequent to brain injury and believed to be consequent to the organic alteration in the cortex resulted from this dual interest in therapy and diagnosis. The two interest areas, however, were rarely collated. The speech pathologist has been concerned almost entirely with the speech problem, while psychologists and psychiatrists investigated over-all behavior and gave only secondary consideration to language disorders.

It is a strongly held conviction of the present writer that maximal success in therapy can only be obtained when it includes due consideration of the personality of the patient and the appearance of behavioral aberrations. Conversely, it is held that complete differential diagnosis can only be made when the language problem is evaluated in all its complex forms. The aphasia therapist must be prepared to recognize behavioral abnormalities when they occur and must be equipped to assist in their resolution when they have a negative effect on therapeusis.

The following sections are devoted to a review of nonlanguage phenomena noted by students of brain disease, as well as those seen by the author in patients who have come under his care.

Early Observations of Nonlanguage Behavior of the Brain-Injured

Marie gave the first adequate description of the nonlanguage behavior of the brain-injured adult. In 1906 he described in detail the problems of attention, memory, and association of ideas common to this group.[1] He was the first to recognize that they were integral and differentiating parts of the disorder. Since then, the range of deviations of behavior that have been reported has extended from the higher intellectual functions described by Halstead[2] and other psychologists to the posttraumatic psychoses described in psychiatric textbooks.[3]

Jackson viewed the aphasic adult as a living entity displaying pathognomonic behavior, saying that "the behavior symptoms we see are positive mental symptoms, survival on a lower level of evolution . . . the illusions, hallucinations, delusions, and extravagant behavior are the outcome of nervous elements on the lower level of evolution remaining."[4] Jackson believed that the behavior of this type of patient was the activity of an individual who had lost the higher and more recently developed intellectual controls. In consequence his behavior had retrogressed. It was only through reorganization of the remaining tissue that there could be a return to normal behavior.

The truth of Jackson's concept of dissolution was seen many times in the behavior of patients reported in the present volume, especially in those who came to the retraining process in a vegetative state. These patients were performing on one of life's lowest levels. The following comment of a neurologist who examined such a patient before his first visit to the De Witt General Hospital Aphasia Center illustrates the point: "Content to sleep at all hours, even find-

---

[1] Pierre Marie, cited by F. Moutier in *L'Aphasie de Broca* (Paris: G. Steinhil, 1908), p. 202: ". . . parfois difficiles à mettre en evidence, mais que l'on peut toujours retrouver. Ce sont des défauts de la mimique, de la mémoire, de l'association des idées . . ." "[they are] sometimes difficult to demonstrate, but [they] can always be found. They are defects of imitation, of memory, of association of ideas. . . ."

[2] Ward C. Halstead, "Behavioral Effects of Lesions of the Frontal Lobes in Man," *Archives of Neurology and Psychiatry*, XLII (October, 1939), 780–83.

[3] Stanley Cobb, *Borderlands of Psychiatry* (Baltimore: The Williams and Wilkins Co., 1941).

[4] Hughlings Jackson, quoted in Samuel J. Beck, *The Rorschach Test: I. Basic Processes* (New York: Grune & Stratton, Inc., 1944), p. 108.

ing it difficult to stay awake for meals. Requiring attention for all bodily acts. Uninterested in the environment. Unmotivated and wandering in attention even when highly stimulated. Lacking fear, anxiety, or tension." [5] At such a time the physiological and psychological behavior seem strangely similar. The patient is at his lowest ebb both in physical and psychological reaction patterns.

Control of Activity by the Frontal Cortex

Until recently the frontal lobe was considered a silent area and no particular function was ascribed to this region of the cortex. However, recent studies indicate that although in this area there may be little focal control of language, there is a wide and vital control of behavior. Frontal lobectomy, introduced by Moniz and elaborated by Freeman and Watts, and the study of the results of operations on humans by Halstead, Hebb, Penfield, and Lashley have greatly extended our knowledge of the controls exercised by this region.[6] The deviations of behavior observed by these writers are almost completely nonlanguage. It is remarkable that similar abnormalities of behavior were seen in almost every subject reported on in the present volume regardless of the site of the injury, whether in the frontal or some other lobe of the cortex.

Halstead has described a framework of behavior related to the frontal lobe derived from his exhaustive testing program. He summarized the factors that he was able to isolate in the following manner:

1. A central integrative field factor C. This factor represents the organized experience of the individual.

2. A factor of abstraction A. This factor concerns the basic capacity to group to a criterion, as in the elaboration of categories, and involves the comprehension of essential similarities and differences. It is the fundamental growth principle of the ego.

3. A power factor P. This factor reflects the undistorted power factor of the brain. It operates to counterbalance or regulate the

---

[5] From confidential United States Army Medical Records on one of the subjects of the present study (see Chapter 5 below).

[6] E. Moniz, cited in W. Freeman and J. W. Watts, *Psychosurgery* (Springfield, Ill.: Charles C. Thomas, Publisher, 1942). Freeman and Watts, *op. cit.* Ward C. Halstead, "Specialization of Behavioral Functions and the Frontal Lobes," in Association for Research in Nervous and Mental Disease, *The Frontal Lobes* (Baltimore: The Williams & Wilkins Co., 1948). D. O. Hebb, "Man's Frontal Lobes," *Archives of Neurology and Psychiatry,* LIV (July, 1945), 10–24. W. Penfield and J. Evans, "The Frontal Lobe in Man," *Brain,* LVIII (April, 1935), 115–33. K. S. Lashley, "Factors Limiting Recovery After Central Nervous System Lesions," *Journal of Nervous and Mental Diseases,* LXXXVIII (October, 1938), 733–55.

affective forces and thus frees the growth principle of the ego for further ego differentiation.

4. A directional factor D. This vector constitutes the medium through which the process factors, noted here, are exteriorized at any given moment.[7]

Halstead has also described the inability of the brain-injured patient to shift from one thought or act to another with the ease of the uninjured, to hold thoughts in mind for consecutive patterning, and to group things in a normal manner.[8]

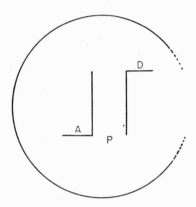

Fig. 1.—"A conceptual model of unit biological intelligence which may variously be reduplicated through the cerebral cortex. Outer ring in figure represents the central integrative factor C. The A (abstraction), P (power), and D (directional or modality) factors diagrammed as being interrelated and collectively related to C." (After Halstead, *Brain and Intelligence,* p. 97.)

These deviations in behavior are also seen frequently in patients who have suffered injuries in regions of the cortex remote from the frontal lobe. Many writers have tried to explain this discrepancy. C. von Monakow formulated his theory of "diachisis," in which he held that abnormal behavior observed after injury to the brain was the result of injury to connecting fibers as well as injury to the local area.[9] Goldstein explains the phenomenon as an "impairment of a function due to the damage of a not directly affected lesion by irritation emanating from a defect at another place."[10]

[7] Ward C. Halstead, *Brain and Intelligence* (Chicago: University of Chicago Press, 1948), p. 147.

[8] Ward C. Halstead, "Preliminary Analysis of Grouping Behavior in Patients with Cerebral Injury," *Journal of Psychology,* XX (May, 1940), 14.

[9] C. von Monakow, *Die Lokalisation in Grosshirn* (Wiesbaden: Bergmann, 1914).

[10] Kurt Goldstein, "Mental Changes Due to Frontal Lobe Damage," *Journal of Psychology,* XVII (April, 1944), 193.

Lashley holds that, "in addition to their specific function, all parts of the cortex exercise a facilitative effect upon the rest." [11] Whatever the correct explanation, it is true that signs ascribed to particular types and locations of injuries do appear in individuals with injuries in other regions. In this volume, no exact behavior pattern is ascribed to any particular region of the cortex. Aberrant behavior does appear after injury, and it may follow damage to any part of the cortex.

Behavior Following Brain Injury.—Freeman and Watts have given an excellent picture of the typical behavior seen after prefrontal lobectomy. "There is progression from a disoriented, apathetic state with little initiative or concern about self or the world, an indifference to society, a slowing of performance, extremely concrete thinking, with poor attention span and a lack of interest in recovery." [12]

Goldstein studied the behavior of soldiers of the German army injured in World War 1. He described the "catastrophic reaction" of the brain-injured adult. He observed that, when such a patient is faced by a problem that frustrates him, he frequently reacts in the following way: "looks dazed, changes color, becomes agitated, anxious, begins to fumble, his pulse may become irregular; a moment before amicable, he is now sullen, evasive, exhibits temper or even becomes aggressive." [13] Goldstein believed that this was the typical behavior of the average normal man when faced by catastrophic events. This pattern has been observed by many students and is now accepted as one of the common behavior abnormalities in aphasia. Since the aphasia therapist continually frustrates the aphasic subject during the recovery process, this behavior must be recognized and dealt with objectively.

Goldstein and a series of collaborators observed the tendency of brain-injured soldiers to think on a concrete level. This observation is of such extreme importance to the therapeutic process that it deserves considerable discussion. The authors wrote that "organic pathology in patients with brain disease disintegrates human behavior in such a way that the capacity to abstract is impaired to greater or lesser degree in every patient. Thus he becomes more or less reduced to a level of concreteness of situational thinking and acting so that he can perform only those tasks which can be fulfilled in a

[11] Lashley, *op. cit.*, p. 744.
[12] Freeman and Watts, *op. cit.*, p. 208.
[13] Kurt Goldstein, *Aftereffects of Brain Injuries in War* (New York: Grune & Stratton, Inc., 1942), p. 70.

concrete manner." [14]   For proof of this contention, the authors presented a series of tests of concept formation.[15]

This theory of the loss of abstracting ability by brain-injured
patients, as demonstrated by the concept formation tests of Goldstein and his collaborators, has become widely accepted. Eisenson,
however, studying the effects of brain injury during the recent war,
points out that "only two of thirty patients especially studied for loss
of capacity to abstract showed any significant loss in this capacity." [16]
In the patients seen by the present writer, twenty of seventy-one had
varying degrees of difficulty on the Goldstein tests at the beginning
of training. When the same subjects were tested at the end of training, only nine of the twenty still showed loss of abstracting ability.
It would seem that loss of the ability to abstract, while frequently
present after head injury, can be reduced by training.

Behavior Characteristics Defined by Tests

In recent years there has been an increase in the use of tests
to collect information on the common behavior manifestations
of the individual after cerebral disease. In the area of projective
tests the most fruitful has been the Rorschach psychodiagnostic or
ink blot test.[17] The leading student of this method of personality
evaluation in the field of intracranial pathology has been Z. A. Piotrowsky. According to him the brain-injured adult shows constriction of personality, slowing down of mental processes, affective
lability or emotional instability, inhibition of spontaneity, repetition
in thought and action, inadequacy, lack of conformity in thought and
behavior, and a tendency toward automatic verbalization.[18] Using
the same test, Beck has reported that the "efficiency of mental processes would vary" in patients with cerebral pathology.[19] Harrower-
Erickson stated in 1940 that in the Rorschach performances of patients with brain tumor their records "show restricted and constricted
personality, extraordinarily uniform when contrasted with the variety

---

[14] Kurt Goldstein and M. Scheerer, "Abstract and Concrete Behavior," *American Psychological Association Monographs*, LI, 9.
    [15] The tests designed and used included: (*a*) cube test, (*b*) color-sorting test,
(*c*) object-sorting test, (*d*) color-form test, and (*e*) stick test. See Goldstein and
Scheerer, *op. cit.*
    [16] Jon Eisenson, "Aphasics: Observations and Tentative Conclusions," *Journal
of Speech Disorders*, XII (September, 1947), 291.
    [17] Hermann Rorschach, *Psychodiagnostik* (Berne: Huber, 1921).
    [18] Z. A. Piotrowsky, "The Rorschach Method and Its Application in Organic
Disturbances of the Central Nervous System," *Rorschach Research Exchange*,
I (1936–37), 23.
    [19] Beck, *op. cit.*, p. 107.

found in normal subjects." [20]   In contrast with these reports of positive findings in the ink blot test is the report by Ackerly and Benton on a case of bilateral frontal lobe defect in which the protocol showed that on "two of the three performances (there was not) a single 'organic' (Piotrowsky) sign. The third performance showed one sign (perseveration). None of Harrower-Erickson's three specific findings is found in any of the Rorschach records." [21]

Intelligence tests, too, have made their contributions to the study of personality aberrations common to the brain-injured adult.   The most productive of these has been the Wechsler-Bellevue test of adult intelligence.   Wechsler in his analysis of the test results of the patients suffering from cerebral disorders says that "disorganization of the intellectual processes [is] observed in most organic brain cases irrespective of type." [22] He lists the following areas in which the subjects of his study showed deviation from the norm:

1. Disturbance in the visual motor field
2. A loss of shift
3. Various memory defects
4. A falling off of capacities involving organization and synthesizing ability
5. Loss of conceptual thinking
6. Rigidity in thought processes
7. Disability in new learning

Malmo reported the results of a battery of twenty-one tests used on seven cases of bilateral frontal gyrectomy and eight cases of bilateral frontal lobotomies. He found among other unrelated factors "a consistent slight drop in general intelligence [and] a significant reduction in vocabulary, in which changes in the direction of greater concreteness of definition were noted postoperatively.

"It was concluded that the balance of evidence at the present time favors interpretation of the observed deficit in terms of reduction in the patient's ability to maintain set in the face of interference." [23]

---

[20] M. R. Harrower-Erickson, "Personality Changes Accompanying Cerebral Lesions," *Archives of Neurology and Psychiatry*, XLIII (1940), 889.

[21] S. S. Ackerly and A. L. Benton, "Report of a Case of Bilateral Frontal Lobe Deficit," in Association for Research in Nervous and Mental Disease, *The Frontal Lobes* (Baltimore: The Williams & Wilkins Co., 1948), p. 494.

[22] David Wechsler, *Measurement of Adult Intelligence* (Baltimore: The Williams & Wilkins Co., 1944), p. 153.

[23] R. H. Malmo, "Psychological Aspects of Frontal Gyrectomy and Frontal Lobotomy in Mental Patients," in Association for Research in Nervous and Mental Disease, *The Frontal Lobes* (Baltimore: The Williams & Wilkins Co., 1948), p. 562.

Observations Made in Army Hospitals

A summary of the most frequently observed behavioral tendencies in the aphasic patients in army hospitals in 1945 was described in a privileged army report on aphasia.[24] Since this report includes observations made on patients whose cases are reported below, it is presented here in considerable detail, although normative data are not available.

The report shows that many patients with cerebral disease had the following behavioral characteristics:

1. Reduced capacity for abstract behavior
2. Disturbances of concentration and attention
3. Memory defects
4. Increased irritability, fatigability, anxiety, euphoria, and various psychosomatic disturbances
5. Reduced ability to adjust to new situations
6. Strong tendency toward perseveration
7. Social withdrawal, shyness, and seclusiveness

These listed characteristics were observations made before the patients were given training. They were not seen in every patient but were common enough to govern a generalized program. The curricula developed in the army centers were to some degree based upon these common findings.

It is to be noted that normative statistical data are lacking for most of the behavioral manifestations mentioned in the preceding paragraphs. As Wendell Johnson pointed out in a personal communication to the author, many of the signs mentioned by such men as Wechsler [25] and Goldstein [26] are to be found in descriptions of the "intellectualizing" behavior of the general population. It is not the fact of their occurrence in the observed behavior of the brain-damaged patient that is important here, but rather the fact that they seem to occur more frequently; in different constellations of behavior, and usually to greater degrees of intensity in this type of patient than in the general population. What is lacking is corroborative controlled research on both the selected, cortically disrupted population and the general population. This poses an important future task for psychologists and neurologists. However, the con-

---

[24] Privileged United States Army Medical Department communication entitled, "Aphasic Language Disorders," October, 1945. No objective data were given in the report.

[25] *Op. cit.*

[26] *Aftereffects of Brain Injuries in War.*

firmation of many of these signs by clinical observation indicates the importance of using these noted common behavior patterns as signposts in the structuring of therapy. If the aberrant behavior is expected and properly handled in therapy today, confirmation by statistical procedures should not be lacking in the future.

Physical Concomitants

Paralysis.—An important area of concern with many brain-injured patients and one that must be considered in planning an over-all therapeusis is that of paralysis of the extremities. A common aftermath of head injury is hemiplegia of the contralateral side of the body. Thus, an individual with an injury to the left side of the brain frequently shows a paralysis or paresis of the extremities of the right side of the body. The frequency of occurrence in the total brain-injured population of such paralysis is not available in medical statistics. In the seventy-one patients reported on in detail in later chapters, however, only four did not show paralysis of some degree. The paralysis noted in the great majority of the patients had a marked effect upon the therapeutic program. It was necessary to develop the therapy around the physical limitations of the patients. The factor of limitation of movement should be borne in mind whenever a therapeutic program is being devised for aphasia. Care must be exercised in providing for physiotherapy, selected occupational therapy, and proper recreational activity. A detailed description of the organization of therapy for aphasic patients has appeared in one of the professional journals.[27]

The author found that anxiety concerning recovery from paralysis was one of the most prominent fixations in his patients. In this regard the tendency of the lower extremity to regain function long before and to a much greater degree than the upper extremity should be noted. Bucy has pointed out the reason for this in an article stating that "removal of the precentral motor cortex from one human hemisphere results in an immediate complete paralysis of the face, arm, and leg of the opposite side. Soon the face will show evidence of recovery, particularly in the upper part. . . . The recovery in the arm is always very limited . . . the leg does much better. . . . This recovery in man is due to innervation from the intact ipsilateral hemisphere." [28]

[27] Joseph Wepman, "Organization of Aphasia Therapy," *Journal of Speech Disorders,* XII (December, 1947), 405–9.

[28] Paul Bucy, "Organization of Central Nervous System Control of Muscular Activity," *Chicago Medical Society Bulletin,* LI (April 30, 1949), 836–66.

In reviewing the data obtained from the intensive study of brain-injured patients reported in a later section, an interesting and possibly exceedingly important factor was noted. In the seventy-one aphasia patients studied, none had a left hemiplegia or hemiparesis. Two of the group were known to have used their left hands exclusively prior to their injuries and had been considered left-handed. Both had right hemiparesis, and both had aphasia. Of the six hundred and ninety-six brain-damaged patients examined at the De Witt General Hospital Aphasia Center, forty-seven had left hemiplegia or hemiparesis and none had residual aphasia. In a further review of data from the author's files, both prewar and afterward, it was noted that not a single case of aphasia had been seen after right brain damage.

The literature on this point is not conclusive. Kussmaul reports that the early neurologists Pye Smith, Hughlings Jackson, and John Ogle claimed that lesions of the right hemisphere in left-handed persons would produce an aphasia.[29] Neither Kussmaul nor the authorities he quotes, however, mention their conclusions in terms of actual patients. The first actual case discussed in the literature was that of a patient of Bastian's in 1898. Here a left-handed, ambidextrous, eighteen-year-old patient who was hemiplegic on the left side was reported as being speechless. This patient came to autopsy shortly thereafter, and the report showed a large area of softening of the right hemisphere. The left hemisphere was noted as being perfectly healthy.[30] No evidence is offered of the intellectual capacity of this patient, nor of the actual time elapsed after the brain trauma before the patient's decease.

German neurologists played a prominent role around the turn of the century in research on brain function. Von Monakow, in his critical discussion of absolute cerebral localization of function,[31] noted the preponderance of the left hemisphere in cortical activity. He was of the opinion that, despite the work on left-handedness by E. Stier, much of the proof for speech centers and right brain function was hypothetical. He argued that belief in the theory that right brain speech centers control language in left-handed people, or that any speech center has absolute control, was developed under the strong influence of the doctrine of specific localization and needed revision. While reviewing case material, he quotes instances of

    [29] A. Kussmaul, cited in F. H. Simon, "Casuistische Beitrige zur lehre von der Aphesie," *Berliner klinische Wochenschrift*, VIII (November, 1871), 537–39.
    [30] H. D. Bastian, *A Treatise on Aphasia* (London: H. K. Lewis, 1898), p. 90.
    [31] C. von Monakow, *Die Lokalisation in Grosshirn* (Wiesbaden: Bergmann, 1914).

"long-lasting word-muteness" in which the left-sided focus was essentially outside of the "third left frontal gyrus." He also commented, without description of the patient's speech, on right-handed individuals in whom grave aphasic disturbances occurred as the result of a "focus in the right hemisphere." It is unfortunate that the status of the left hemisphere in the patient was not discussed.

Oppenheim in 1913 discussed the German literature on the concept that speech centers of the left-handed person are located in areas of the right hemisphere corresponding to the centers in the left hemisphere in right-handed. He mentions ". . . a few cases [which] have been described by Bastian and Dickinson in which left-handed persons were attacked by aphasia and right hemiplegia due to a focal lesion in the left hemisphere . . . exceptionally, as Bramwell thinks, it may happen that in a right-handed person the right hemisphere contains the speech centers and vice versa. Spiller (*Review of Neurology*, 1906) reports about a case that was interpreted in this sense. I have together with Heine observed a case which cannot be interpreted otherwise: a lesion in the occipito-temporal region of the right hemisphere in a right-handed person had produced optic aphasia which disappeared after removing the pus. (Heine, *Deutsche medizinische Wochenschrift*, 1903.)"[32]

Oppenheim went on to say that "particularly in tumors of the right frontal and temporal lobes aphasic disturbances have repeatedly been described. Joffroy (*Revue Neurologique*, 1903) believes that this happens in persons who were born left-handed and had become right-handed only by education; other experiences speak against this assumption. Word-deafness due to a lesion in the right lobus temporalis is further described by Mollard (*Lyon Medicine*, 1903). Senator saw aphasia with left hemiplegia due to an embolic softening of the right temporal lobe in a right-handed person. I, too, know two corresponding cases." Additional German literature is referred to by Oppenheim on this same point,[33] but no case studies are cited.

Zollinger reported the only known case of the removal of a total left cerebral hemisphere in 1935.[34] The patient, a female aged forty-three years, was aphasic before operation. Afterward she was taught to say a few words and could use them with some accuracy.

[32] H. Oppenheim, *Nervous Diseases* (Berlin: Karger, 1913).

[33] E. Weber, *Ursachen und Folgen der recht Shaendigkeit* (Halle, 1905); Dinkler, in *Archiv für Psychiatrie*, XLII; Le Fort, *Thèse de Paris* (1903); M. Meyer, in *Deutsche medizinische Wochenschrift*, 1909; Stier, in *Neurologische Zentralblatt*, 1909; Souques, in *Revue Neurologique*, 1910; Mingazzini, in *Nouvelle Iconographie*, 1910; Dejerine-Thomas, in *Revue Neurologique*, 1912.

[34] R. Zollinger, "Removal of Left Cerebral Hemisphere," *Archives of Neurology and Psychiatry*, XXXIV (November, 1935), 1055.

The vocabulary was limited but believed to be purposive. The patient died on the seventeenth postoperative day. While this is not a conclusive case, it strongly suggests that the right hemisphere was beginning to take over the language function.

In 1936 Chesher commented on two left-handed patients with aphasia following removal of brain tumors from the right cerebral hemisphere.[35] In a personal communication Dr. Chesher had this to say about the language problem in these patients: "The two patients cited were left-handed and had lesions in the language zone of the right hemisphere; both were aphasic. Both individuals had tumors; one was operated, and the other was examined in autopsy. The latter patient's aphasic picture fluctuated during his clinical course but was characterized primarily by a jargon aphasia. The other patient's lesion was more forward and his disability was essentially that of a dysarthria." These findings are in keeping with the present writer's observations. Language disturbances of the right-brain-damaged patient fall in the area of language skill as dysarthric manifestations rather than aphasic problems of reception or production. Jargon aphasia is most commonly seen either in the immediate posttraumatic period or in the patient with widespread intellectual deficit.

Nielsen reports the case of a "banker aged sixty-eight years [who] was born left-handed, but trained from the age of eight to write with the right hand . . . he suffered a cerebral thrombosis with left hemiplegia and complete aphasia from which he recovered in a few weeks except for a mild hemiparesis."[36] This pattern is frequently observed—the immediate aphasia following brain damage of any kind, which clears spontaneously during the immediate posttraumatic period.

In the two large studies published since the recent war, Luria's investigation of 394 brain-injured patients in Moscow[37] and Butfield and Zangwill's research on 70 patients in England,[38] not one case of right brain damage and aphasia was noted.

The author had the opportunity recently to discuss this same problem with the language investigator of the Montreal Neurological Institute. At that institution, where the effects of brain damage upon

[35] E. C. Chesher, "Some Observations Concerning the Relation of Handedness to the Language Mechanism," *Bulletin of the Neurological Institute of New York,* IV (April, 1936), 557.

[36] J. M. Nielsen, "The Cortical Motor Pattern Apraxias," in Association for Research in Nervous and Mental Disease, *The Frontal Lobes,* p. 573.

[37] Alexander Luria, "Topical Syndromes of Traumatic Aphasia," unpublished manuscript loaned by Helen Black, literary agent of the U.S.S.R., New York.

[38] E. Butfield and O. Zangwill, "Re-education in Aphasia," *Journal of Neurology, Neurosurgery and Psychiatry,* IX, New Series, No. 2 (April, 1946), 75–79.

language have been carefully noted for many years, only two cases of right cerebral injury and subsequent communication deficit have been seen. On examination of the records of these patients it was noted that dysarthria rather than aphasia was the outstanding symptom in one, while the other showed a mixed language problem which could not be identified, but could not be classified as an aphasia.

The immediate conclusions to be drawn from this observed material, which seems to deny an old and strongly held postulate concerning cortical function, are twofold: first, that language deficits following damage to the right hemisphere either are of the nature of dysarthrias or, if aphasic-like, last only a short time and are overcome spontaneously; second, that permanent aphasia, the propositionalizing disorder of symbolization in language, occurs only after injury to the left cerebral hemisphere, regardless of cortical dominance.

If further observation and research should bear out the hypotheses stated, the implications appear to be far-reaching and important.

Convulsions.—One other important physical concomitant of brain injury is the traumatic convulsive seizure. This factor is so well known that lengthy discussion of it here is not indicated. The effects of the appearance of seizures upon the patient, upon his attitude toward self and his attitude toward recovery, must, however, be recognized and adequately covered during therapy. The writer has seen aphasic patients develop a marked withdrawal from society and from therapy as the result of the appearance of an unexplained single seizure. Only by preparation of the patient prior to the event has it been possible to avoid these debilitating withdrawal symptoms. In this regard it is suggested that the therapist be cognizant of the growing body of knowledge concerning convulsions. Since World War II, with the development of new medications for the control of seizures, the advancements made by neurosurgeons in removing irritative forces that produce convulsions, and the progress made through electroencephalography in defining and localizing the epileptoid foci, the future of the patient with convulsions is becoming vastly improved.[39]

---

[39] The student in this area may be referred to: *Journal of Electroencephalography and Neurophysiology;* Association for Research in Nervous and Mental Disease, *Epilepsy* (Baltimore: The Williams & Wilkins Co., 1947) ; W. Penfield and T. C. Erickson, *Epilepsy and Cerebral Localization* (Springfield, Ill.: Charles C. Thomas, Publisher, 1941).

Synthesis of Observed Nonlanguage Manifestations

The commonly seen behavior mechanisms reported seem to be the result of two major etiological factors: first, those directly attributable to the brain damage (these should be considered as primary, that is, reducible only by a resolution of the disorder or a reintegration of function in the cortex); second, those signs which appear as the patient attempts to regain his ego integrity and struggles with the inadequacy of his nonintegrated cerebral structure. Undoubtedly, any attempt to draw a line between these two groups would be arbitrary and not too meaningful. There appears unquestionably to be a suggestion of disordered soma underlying all the behavior, while a secondary psychological effect follows each facet of behavior directly traceable to disintegration of brain tissue. The aphasia therapist should be aware of the dichotomous tendency of these observed signs, indicating the irreversible nature of cortical tissue destruction as well as the residual psychological changes.

Table 1 shows the most frequently observed behavioral manifestations. Some, but not all, were seen by the author in the patients under his care. Others are included because of the consistency with which they appear in the literature, even though they lack personal confirmation.

Changing Personality Characteristics.—The aphasia therapist must recognize the changing nature of the behavior of the brain-injured patient. In almost no other disability is as much inconsistency of behavior to be noted. While in the protected environments, the hospital or the home, where most things are ordered and provided for the patient, it would be expected that his behavior would be comparatively stable. This is frequently not the case, however. Mood swings of depression varied by euphoria are common, while even specific behavior mechanisms vary from day to day and from morning to evening. At times the patient will be seen to be easily frustrated and impulsive in his reaction to very simple external stimuli. At other times he will appear to be thoughtful, considerate, and maximally cooperative. The therapist must recognize these shifting patterns. The utmost use must be made of the periods of maximal cooperation while stimulation should be kept minimal during the opposite periods. In terms of the over-all therapeusis it must be remembered that the patient changes through a process of internal readjustment and externally induced learning. Each step he takes along the road towards recovery brings a whole series of new percep-

TABLE 1

NONLANGUAGE DEVIATIONS IN APHASIA

1. Loss of attention and concentration
2. Loss of memory
3. Reduced association of ideas
4. Abstract-concrete imbalance (loss of ability to abstract; concrete concept formation)
5. Poor organizing ability
6. Poor judgment
7. Perseveration
8. Constriction of thought and interest
9. Reduced ability to generalize, categorize, group, or plan future action
10. Reduced general level of intelligence
11. Reduced ability to inhibit internal emotional forces which disturb the action of the intellect (Halstead's "power factor")
12. Inability to shift
13. Psychomotor retardation
14. Feelings of inadequacy
15. Egocentricity
16. Increased irritability and fatigability
17. Euphoria
18. Social withdrawal and seclusiveness
19. Reduced ability to adjust to new situations
20. Catrastrophic reactions
21. Reduced initiative
22. Disinterest in the environment, both physical and human
23. Externalization of behavior; a lack of introspection or self-criticism
24. Reduced spontaneity
25. Perplexity (a distrust of one's own ability)
26. Automatic verbalization
27. Impulsive behavior
28. Regressive, infantile behavior
29. Impotence (the inability to correct behavior one knows is wrong)
30. Posttraumatic psychotic behavior showing illusions, hallucinations, delusions, and extravagant behavior
31. Anxiety and tension
32. Convulsive seizures
33. Changing personality profile, the emergence and submergence of characteristics
34. Hemiplegia

tions to him. Each change makes the patient a new and different person. Recognition of these changes by the patient are of extreme importance for they serve as can no other force as motivation towards continuation of therapy.

The concept of change in the patient is to be seen in still another light. Often when therapy begins soon after trauma, the patient may appear to be in a state that is best described as vegetative. During the first months, and in many patients during the very first posttraumatic days, he may go through very rapid physical and psychological changes. During this time contact and equilibrium are being regained in a world in which he has been nonexistent for all practical purposes. Viewed at one time by the therapist, he may show little reason to hope for recovery, while a short time later the prognosis may seem infinitely improved. These dramatic changes are almost always limited to the immediate posttraumatic period.

Butfield and Zangwill have referred to this early period as the stage of "spontaneous recovery." [40] Luria has also paid considerable attention to the same period in a recent manuscript, even entitling one of his chapters "Dynamics of Aphasic Syndromes at Successive Stages of the Traumatic Disease of the Cerebrum." [41] It is Luria's belief that there are two distinct stages of recovery. He called the first period the "initial stage," where both permanent and temporary language and personality deviation processes are observed. The second period, after the first six months has elapsed, he called the "residual stage," where only persistent language and personality problems could be observed. Luria indicated in his study that of 394 patients, 43 per cent showed "residual" signs which would require re-education or psychotherapy. The other patients recovered spontaneously within the "initial" period. In Chapter 6 below, data are given on the effects of therapy when started soon after trauma as compared with the effects of training when started later.

The aphasia therapist must at all times be aware of these changing facets of the problem he is treating. He must not expect to see consistency of behavior, but rather must expect a constantly shifting picture. Most of the observed manifestations reported in the preceding sections were subject to these variations, even though they were described as pathognomonic of the behavior of the brain-injured patient.

Summary

The implications to be derived from recognition of common behavioral mechanisms after intracranial pathology are far-reaching and important. An over-all therapeutic design which failed to take them into account would be unrealistic and doomed to failure. The very multiplicity of different abnormalities indicates the wide variety of behavior which can be expected and the consequent need of careful psychological training for the therapist.

It is axiomatic to say that language therapy without psychotherapy is futile and often harmful in itself, for the aphasic patient

---

[40] Op. cit.
[41] Op. cit.

who has recovered language but has not resolved his behavioral adjustmental problems must be considered an unsuccessfully treated patient. The ultimate goal of therapy must be the ability to function properly in society. Without resolution of the aberrant behavior noted, readjustment for the brain-injured patient can only mean a continued life as either a recluse or an object of social disapproval.

Chaper 4

CLASSIFICATION AND NOMENCLATURE
OF APHASIA SYMPTOMS

As interest grew in the study of cortical function, new concepts developed, new language areas were isolated, and new methods of classifying brain-damaged patients were evolved. Each researcher had his own ideas concerning the names that should be used to identify the different types of language problems. As a result, no consistent classification of aphasic disorders ever developed. The aphasia therapist studying previous research and theoretical opinion in the literature is easily confounded by the welter of overlapping categories and neologistic terms. To clarify this muddled picture somewhat, the following sections present a review of the more prominent classification principles found in the literature. As will be seen, certain basic or fundamental concepts stand out. These form the structure for the classification method and major technical nomenclature adapted for the present work.

Traditional Concepts of Nomenclature

Broca gave the name *aphémie* to the language problem which he first described.[1] This was a word that he drew from the Greek word meaning "without speech." A year later Trousseau, one of Broca's teachers, remarked that the word was used improperly. He agreed that the coined word *aphémie* could represent "without speech," but pointed out that in Greek it also meant "infamy." Trousseau suggested the word *aphasie,* from the Greek word for "speechlessness." This word he believed would be more apt and less confusing.[2]

Broca, it appears, was unable to attend the meeting at which Trousseau made this comment, but in an untitled letter to the *Gazette des Hôpitaux* he defended his choice of words both eloquently and logically. Then, because it evidently meant little to him which word

---

[1] Paul Broca, "Rémarques Sur le siège de la faculté du langage articulé suivé d'une observation d'aphémie," *Bulletin Société Anatomique de Paris,* XXVI, 2me série (August, 1861), 327–31.

[2] A. Trousseau, "De l'Aphasie," *Clinique Médical,* XXXV, 1st series (1862), 22–23.

was used, he agreed to the use of the word aphasie.[3] The manner of Broca's acceptance appeared to incense Trousseau. He wrote an immediate, angry, and very lengthy reply, which appeared in the next issue of the same journal. He entitled his response "De l'aphasie, maladie décrite récemment sous le nom impropre d'Aphémie." [4] Through the insistence of Trousseau and the unconcern of Broca, the word aphasie, or in English, aphasia, meaning speechlessness, became a fixed word in a field which now recognizes that the very act it describes is only one of many language disorders which arise as the result of injury to the brain.

Classification by Function of the Nervous System

Wernicke distinguished the aphasia he first described from that described by Broca by the part of the nervous system that he believed affected. Wernicke spoke of *sensory* and *motor* aphasia and recognized that one involved the receptive and the other the productive side of language.[5] Since that time, the words *sensory* and *motor* have been used to denote at least the general area of function affected. When Arnold Pick later described the aphasia he had seen, he used the descriptive words "expressive" for the motor disturbance and "impressive" for the sensory.[6] Both of these words are used today by many authors. Later writers substituted the word "receptive" for Pick's "impressive" category, and this term is used in Weisenburg and McBride's classification system. These latter authors differentiated four groups of aphasia, as follows:

1. Mixed expressive-receptive
2. Predominantly expressive
3. Predominantly receptive
4. Amnesic [7]

This was the first recognition in the literature of the clinical observation that aphasia is never purely expressive or receptive. For purposes of strict classification, this qualification or preciseness seems to be unnecessary, once it is agreed that pure expressive or receptive difficulties rarely if ever exist. The term "amnesic aphasia" was

---

[3] Paul Broca, untitled open letter, *Gazette des Hôpitaux,* XXXVII (October, 1864), 35 ff.

[4] *Gazette des Hôpitaux,* XXXVIII (November, 1864), 62–63.

[5] C. Wernicke, cited in T. Weisenburg and K. McBride, *Aphasia* (New York: The Commonwealth Fund, Division of Publications, 1935), p. 12.

[6] A. Pick, cited in J. M. Nielsen, *Agnosia, Apraxia, Aphasia* (rev. ed.; New York: Paul B. Hoeber, Inc., Medical Book Department of Harper & Bros., 1946).

[7] *Op. cit.,* p. 82.

not original with Weisenburg and McBride, for Broca recognized its existence many years before. He used the term *verbal amnesics* for those patients who seemed to have little motor difficulty but considerable disability in memory for words. He believed that their difficulty lay in their inability to recall previously learned verbalizations.[8] Apparently, however, Broca conceived aphasia as being largely a motor disability, for he did not include the concept of the sensory defect in his classification system.

Goldstein distinguished three motor or expressive aphasias and, in a less well-organized way, four sensory or receptive types. Of the former he believed there were: "(1) Cortical Aphasias, in which there is a spread of disability affecting the entire cortex; (2) Transcortical Aphasias, in which the defect lies between the sensory and the motor areas; and (3) Subcortical Aphasias, in which the defect is localized and separates an area subserving a particular function from the rest of the cortex. On the sensory side he suggested: (1) Pure word deafness, an inability to comprehend and integrate auditory stimuli; (2) Cortical Sensory Aphasia, in which there is a widespread inability to integrate stimuli from any modality; (3) Central Aphasia, which corresponds to the transcortical type on the motor side and which is frequently referred to as Transcortical Sensory Aphasia; and (4) Amnesic Aphasia, in which the patient cannot use his power of recall." [9]

Sigmund Freud made two contributions to the nomenclature of aphasia. It was Freud's belief that all aphasia was the result of a defect in the conducting mechanism of the cortex and that all aphasia should properly be called *conduction aphasia*.[10] While this seems an oversimplification there is truth in the concept that aphasia has its origin in the associative mechanism and in neural connecting pathways. Freud was more interested, however, in defining the behavior of the aphasic patient than in nomenclature and did not stress his point. Little attention has been paid to this concept of Freud's, although the truth of his assertion has never been contested.

Names of Isolated Functions

Jackson also made a contribution to the naming aspect of the problem of aphasia. He recognized that certain patients talked a language all their own, which was gibberish to the auditor but ap-

---

[8] Broca, "Rémarques Sur le siège de la faculté du langage . . . ," p. 330.
[9] K. Goldstein, cited in Weisenburg and McBride, *Aphasia,* p. 56.
[10] S. Freud, cited in Nielsen, *Agnosia, Apraxia, Aphasia,* p. 7.

parently had some meaning to the speaker. This manifestation he called *jargon aphasia*.[11] Jackson used the term not to distinguish a separate type of aphasia but to describe a peculiar and outwardly meaningless language form.

Two other terms, *agnosia* and *apraxia,* are widely used in the literature. The former, suggested originally by Freud, means loss of the function of recognition of individual sensory stimuli.[12] "Apraxia" has been attributed to many writers, although the first important mention of the word is found in H. Liepmann's analysis of a case in 1900.[13] Apraxia is defined as the inability to perform particular muscular movements because of cortical difficulty. These terms are rarely used alone, but are accompanied by descriptive adjectives indicating the particular receptive or expressive functions affected. Thus, Liepmann spoke of "apraxia of the speech muscles," [14] and Gerstmann's syndrome is called *Fingeragnosie*.[15]

Modern Nomenclatures

Recognizing that none of the existing nomenclatures could express his precise anatomical and clinical observations, Nielsen developed a system of his own. He describes his observations of each patient in the following terms:

1. Type of disorder (agnosia, apraxia, aphasia)
2. Anatomical location of the associated intracranial injury (frontal, parietal, etc.)
3. Modality affected (visual, auditory, etc.)
4. Function affected (reading, writing, etc.) [16]

The classification results in a four-part description. For example, such a classification as "Agnosia, visual, angular, literal" [17] describes the loss of power to recognize letters by vision alone, because of a lesion in the angular gyrus. Nielsen also believes that a new term is needed for the commonly used *amnesia* and suggests the use of *irreminiscence*. He speaks of a disorder as "Irreminiscence, visual, musical, angular," [18] in describing a case with loss of ability to

---

[11] Hughlings Jackson, "Hughlings Jackson on Aphasia, Edited by Henry Head," *Brain,* XXXVIII (1915), 36.
[12] S. Freud, cited in Weisenburg and McBride, *Aphasia,* p. 101.
[13] H. Liepmann, cited in Weisenburg and McBride, *Aphasia,* p. 37.
[14] H. Liepmann, cited in Nielsen, *Agnosia, Apraxia, Aphasia,* p. 80.
[15] J. Gerstmann, cited in Weisenburg and McBride, *Aphasia,* pp. 59–60.
[16] Nielsen, *op. cit.,* p. 258 ff.
[17] *Ibid.,* p. 251.
[18] Nielsen, *op. cit.,* p. 262.

recall musical notes visually because of an injury in the angular gyrus. His classification system lists eighty-seven different types.

Another contemporary classification system was devised by Luria. This Russian psychologist used a terminology related to his concepts of the basic and intermediate zones of speech. He uses a mixture of traditional definitions, anatomical descriptions and new topographical terms. For example, he speaks of "Residual Aphasia, Wernicke, affecting the basic zone in the fronto-parietal region." [19] Luria's work is new in this country, and his findings on aphasia are as yet unpublished. His classification system and new concepts of the disorder of aphasia have received little critical evaluation.

Henry Pieron, one of the French successors to Broca, returns to the work of another French neurologist, Charcot, for the terminology he uses in his monograph.[20] While adhering for the most part to the classical concepts of Broca and Wernicke, he organizes his data as follows:

1. Verbal Aphasia, an isolated disorder of the verbal comprehension of graphic signs
2. Verbal Deafness, an isolated disorder in which the ability to understand words is lost without disturbance of the peripheral auditory mechanism
3. Aphemia, a disorder in which the language is understood, mental reading is perfect, and mimicry and writing are substituted for oral expression
4. Agraphia, a disorder in which the ability to write is lost.[21]

Pieron believes that these four disabilities can be observed in many cases of aphasia, either in an isolated form or as a part of a symptom complex.

The following table lists the most important terms appearing in the literature and the author that first used each one.

Nomenclature Adopted in This Book

Certain basic factors concerning aphasia stand out in considering the need for a classification system. First, there may be a deficit which is primarily in the reception of language; second, the lan-

---

[19] A. Luria, "Essay on the Theory of Traumatic Aphasias," unpublished MS. loaned by Jacob Heiman, editor, *The American Review of Soviet Medicine,* New York, p. 41.

[20] Henri Pieron, *Thought and Brain* (London: Kegan Paul, Trench, Trubner & Co., 1927).

[21] Pieron, *op. cit.,* p. 165.

TABLE 2

MAJOR CONTRIBUTIONS TO THE NOMENCLATURE OF APHASIA
NOTED IN THE LITERATURE

Author	Terms Referring to Expressive Functions	Terms Referring to Receptive Functions
Broca...............	Aphemia	Verbal amnesia
Trousseau.............	Aphasia	Aphasia
Wernicke.............	Motor	Sensory
Pick.................	Expressive	Impressive
Goldstein.............	Subcortical	Pure word deafness
	Transcortical	Sensory, cortical
	Cortical	Central
Kleist................	Speech-sound-muteness	Word-sound-deafness
	Word-muteness	Word-deafness
	Name-muteness	Name-deafness
	Sentence-muteness	Sentence-deafness
Henschen.............	Broca's aphasia	Wernicke's aphasia
	Amusia	Amusia
	Acalculia	Acalculia
	Alexia	Alexia
Freud................	Conduction	Conduction agnosia
Jackson..............	Jargon	Jargon
Weisenburg-McBride.....	Predominantly expressive	Predominantly receptive
Nielsen...............	Aphasia, apractic	Aphasia, visual
	Apraxia, cortical	Agnosia, visual
Pieron...............	Agraphia	Verbal-blindness
Wernicke, Pick..........	Total aphasia	Total aphasia
Weisenburg-McBride.....	Mixed expressive-receptive aphasia	Mixed expressive-receptive aphasia

guage problem may be almost exclusively in the production area; third, there may be a mixture of both areas to such a degree that neither receptive nor productive terms adequately describe the conditions; fourth, some patients show no discernible residuum of language; fifth, the term aphasia itself describes a generalized language disorder, while many of the deficits noted seem to be specific to particular functions.

Recognizing these factors and borrowing from the literature, the author adopted the following classification for use in this book:

1. *Expressive aphasia:* symptoms predominantly motor or productive in nature and consisting of an inability to express ideas through spoken or written language symbols. (After Weisenburg and McBride.)

2. *Receptive aphasia:* symptoms predominantly sensory or receptive in nature and consisting of a disturbance in the ability to com-

prehend language through spoken or written symbols. (After Weisenburg and McBride.)

3. *Expressive-receptive aphasia:* approximately an equal disturbance of both areas. (After Weisenburg and McBride.)

4. *Global aphasia:* all language forms seriously affected to the degree that it is impossible to use one of the preceding categories.

5. *Agnosia:* loss of ability to recognize objects or symbols through a particular sensory channel such as vision or hearing (the loss tends to be specific for words, syllables, letters or other perceptual symbolic units).

6. *Apraxia:* loss of ability to execute simple voluntary acts (the loss tends to be specific for elementary units of action in the expression of language).[22]

These definitions and categories have been used in the manner indicated in the examples shown below:

CASE No. 12. *Expressive Aphasia.* Including a writing apraxia (agraphia), verbal apraxia, number apraxia, and a visual word agnosia (alexia). There was an inability to speak in response to auditory or visual stimuli; an inability to read orally, although some ability to select letters from the written page remained; an inability to write in response to spoken or written stimuli; difficulty in spelling; inability to use numbers either by rote or in problem situations.

CASE No. 41. *Expressive-receptive Aphasia.* Manifested by difficulty in all language spheres. The ability to comprehend simple language commands was retained. No difficulty was seen in the ability to trace forms that did not convey an immediate symbolic meaning. There was also a retained ability to use gestures with meaning and apparent feeling.

CASE No. 18. *Receptive Aphasia.* Including difficulty in comprehending verbal and graphic symbols. Language is present in a very limited degree. Perseveration without self-correction is noted. Mild verbal apraxia is present. The ability to follow gestures is retained.

CASE No. 24. *Global Aphasia.* Manifested by an almost complete inability to comprehend language at any level and a total absence of meaningful expression either verbal or graphic. Some ability to imitate is noted. Jargon is present to a marked degree.

This classification system combines the direct categorization into rough groups determined by the over-all language picture and a discursive description of language behavior. It has the advantage of providing the basis for the beginning of therapy. In a later chapter dealing with examination, the use of the classification system adopted will be further demonstrated.

---

[22] Ward C. Halstead and Joseph M. Wepman, *Manual for the Halstead-Wepman Aphasia Screening Test* (Chicago: Departments of Medicine, Surgery, and Psychology, University of Chicago, 1949).

PART II

RESEARCH FINDINGS DURING WORLD WAR II

Chapter 5

EFFECTS OF TRAINING ON APHASICS

Studies made on brain-injured patients after World War I permitted for the first time the evaluation of considerable numbers of patients in the light of the then current interest in cerebral function and diagnosis. With the upsurge of generalized interest in rehabilitation during and after the more recent war, attention was focused on recovery primarily and only secondarily upon diagnosis and organization of the function of the cortex. The author had an unprecedented opportunity to study the recovery process in a group of seventy brain-injured adults. The findings obtained serve as a basis for the comments in later chapters on therapy and the therapist.

Certain highly important questions were unanswered by the results of previous research. For example, the basic question of the amenability of the aphasic patient to planned therapy had never been discussed. While training for aphasia has been mentioned in the literature as far back as the Mills report of 1906,[1] little or no attention had been paid to it in a systematic way. Many neurologists have held the opinion even in recent years that little can be done for the patient suffering from aphasia.[2] To answer this most fundamental question the research reported in the following pages was conceived and the data were collected. As will be seen in the following chapter, other questions collateral to the first were raised and data applying to them extracted from the material gathered.

Background of the Research Reported in This Book

Several background areas, such as the location of the center where the work was done, the physical structure of the center itself, the staff employed, the selection of subjects for research, and some of the pertinent vital statistics concerning the patients, are presented below.

---

[1] Charles K. Mills, "Treatment of Aphasia by Training," *Journal of the American Medical Association*, XLIII (May, 1904), 1940–49.

[2] Israel Wechsler, *Textbook of Clinical Neurology* (Philadelphia: W. B. Saunders Co., 1939).

Location of Establishment.—The research was carried out at the Aphasia Center established by the United States Army Medical Department in the Ninth Service Command. For the first year (January, 1945, through December, 1945), the center was located at De Witt General Hospital, Auburn, California. From January, 1946, through August, 1946, the center was located at Letterman General Hospital, San Francisco, California.

Physical Equipment.—At De Witt General Hospital, the Center occupied a specially built wing of a new building, the construction of which was in part according to the design established by the writer.[3] This building contained the administrative offices, psychological testing rooms, individual training rooms, large classrooms, and a specially designed occupational therapy room. Adjacent and connected to the Center was another series of offices for social service interviews.

Each classroom was equipped with easel blackboards designed in such a way that the subject seated in a wheel chair could use them without difficulty. There were also special writing boards and mirrors for self-corrective work. In conjunction with the rest of the neuropsychiatric department of the hospital, there was available to the staff a well-equipped library. The Center was located at the end of a ramp upon which the wards housing head-injured patients were situated, so that access to the Center could be had without leaving a covered and sheltered passageway.

For the last six months at Letterman General Hospital, to which the Center moved after the closing of its former location, the structural setup was considerably changed. Here the Center did more than provide educational space. It also housed the subjects. A complete ward was turned over to the Center for its training purposes. In this ward the subjects lived and had their classes, their own occupational therapy shop, and their own recreational facilities. They left the ward for physiotherapy, outdoor recreation, and social activities. While the classrooms were not as well furnished or as numerous as at De Witt General Hospital, the opportunity to observe the behavior of the subjects at all times was of extreme importance.

The Staff.—The Aphasia Center's immediate staff at De Witt General Hospital consisted of four psychologists, three social workers, and four instructors selected from army ranks and trained for

---

[3] Joseph Wepman, "Organization of Aphasia Therapy," *Journal of Speech and Hearing,* XII (December, 1947), 405–9.

their specific duties by the writer. Two of the instructors were qualified speech pathologists. Four competent and experienced civilian teachers were secured from the faculty of Placer Junior College. When the Aphasia Center moved to San Francisco, four other instructors were hired through civil service to replace them. The army also secured the services of two experienced officers, one a speech pathologist and the other a clinical psychologist, who served as assistant directors at the Center at various times, under the direction of the author. The entire staff was given an intensive four-week course in problems common to brain-injured adults. This course covered not only the subject matter to be taught but also the emotional and educational problems that the author thought important to anyone who had not worked with this type of handicapped individual.

In addition to the direct staff of the Center, and adding considerably to the final results achieved, were the following groups: (a) American Red Cross recreational workers; (b) the physiotherapists responsible for muscle re-education; (c) the occupational therapists, about whom much more will be said in a later section; (d) the physical training section of the army hospital in which the Center was located; and (e) the volunteer workers from the many local organizations who did so much to maintain morale among the subjects.

The Center had the opportunity to and did consult with neurological, neurosurgical, and psychiatric medical specialists on problems in their fields.

The training program for the Center's staff covered the following areas:

1. Neuroanatomy and neurology of the brain and the effects of injury upon it; physical effects of epileptiform convulsions; delimitations of paralysis; prognosis for paralyzed patients. (This section was taught by Dr. M. Sall, Chief of the Neurology Section of De Witt General Hospital.)

2. Psychogenic concomitants of brain injury; methods of handling personality deviations; observations on posttraumatic psychosis and usual effects of that disorder upon the individual. (This area was covered by the Chief of the Neuropsychiatric Section of De Witt General Hospital, Dr. Daniel J. Sullivan.)

3. Changes in behavior seen in previous brain-injured patients; etiology of aphasia; classification system for different types of aphasia as reviewed from the literature (see pages 41 and 42); types of language disorders to be expected; use to be made of

different disciplines involved in the re-education process; types of therapy found useful in earlier treatment of aphasia; total program to be developed at the Center. (This area was taught by the writer.)

Procedure of the Aphasia Center

Selection of Subjects.—Every brain-injured patient entering the neurological service of the general hospital in which the Aphasia Center was located was referred for examination.

These patients were given the Sall-Wepman organic screening test [4] by one of the staff psychologists. The results of this test, which measures all the language functions, as well as intellectual deterioration *due to brain injury,* were discussed in conference between the clinical psychologist and the head of the Center. If the presence of language defect was observed on the test protocol, the patient was asked to return to the Center for further testing.

On the second visit to the Center the following testing procedures were used. For an estimation of the patient's intellectual capacity the Wechsler-Bellevue test of adult intelligence was administered. For those patients showing considerable language loss and consequent difficulty with the verbal portion of the test, only the performance portions were given.[5] An estimate of intelligence based upon this test was recorded. It was accepted as the best available method of estimating intellectual capacity for these subjects, although the writer recognized the many weaknesses inherent in making this type of estimate.

The Wechsler-Bellevue scale was adopted mainly because it possessed one highly desirable feature. The test has separate performance and verbal sections, and an I.Q. can be established from either part. For the testing of the subjects before training, the performance section was used alone. After training, the complete test was administered. While many tests measure nonverbal intelligence and show higher correlation coefficients with verbal intelligence tests, the Wechsler-Bellevue is the only one, to the writer's knowledge, that permits discrete scores in performance and verbal areas. Since

---

[4] M. Sall and J. Wepman, "A Screening Survey of Organic Impairment," *Journal of Speech Disorders,* X (May, 1945), 283–86.

[5] David Wechsler, *Measurement of Adult Intelligence* (Baltimore: The Williams & Wilkins Co., 1944), p. 135. Wechsler reports correlation coefficients for the performance portion of his test and Stanford-Binet Form *L* 1937 of + .56 and with the Stanford-Binet 1916 Edition of + .73. The test is divided into two discrete parts, each giving an estimate of intelligence. The correlation of the two parts is stated as + .83, ±.018.

the statistical relationship between the two parts is known, the re-test possibilities were felt to be enhanced.

To estimate the type of language disorder shown by the patients, the Halstead aphasia screening test [6] was administered by the writer. This test was designed to screen language functions of every kind. From the results of the test it was possible to arrive at a gross differential diagnosis of the type of language disorder. This was done for every patient.

The results of the two tests given were discussed in conference. If the magnitude of the problems presented by the patient were such as to necessitate re-education of any type, the patient was referred to the Aphasia Center for training. A study conference was called and attended by the staff of the Center. The findings were reviewed and a tentative working diagnosis was made. The patient was then assigned for training to a particular teacher or group of teachers. A social worker was assigned to study the background material and to contact the family of the subject. A speech pathologist was assigned to assist in the speech training if it was indicated. The ward officer in charge of the patient was notified of the results of the conference, and the patient was placed in the group awaiting training in his ward.

The following criteria were used to determine which of the patients seen at the study level were to be considered as subjects of the present study:

1. Language problems sufficiently severe to require a total program of re-education [7]
2. If in need of immediate training, received injuries six months (or more) before being admitted to training [8]

Thus patients injured at least six months before beginning training, whose aphasias were severe enough to warrant re-education in speech performance, reading, writing, spelling, and mathematics were selected as subjects of the present study.

Population from Which Subjects Were Selected.—As part of the regular examination procedure, every brain-injured patient entering the hospital was studied in the Aphasia Center. Table 3 shows

---

[6] Ward C. Halstead, *Aphasia Screening Test* (Chicago: University of Chicago), distributed personally by the author—experimental copy. A revision of this test by Halstead and Wepman is discussed at length in Chapter 9.

[7] As indicated in Table 3, many patients were seen who needed training in only one or two areas.

[8] See page 34 for a discussion of the reasons for eliminating from the study those patients whose training was begun before the end of the sixth posttraumatic month.

the distribution of cortical disorders examined and the number of individuals who presented an aphasia as part of their disability:

TABLE 3

ANALYSIS OF NEUROPATHOLOGY PRESENTED BY PATIENTS SEEN

Type of Disorder	Aphasia		No Aphasia	Totals
	Initial	Residual *		
Head injury..............	216	69	396	681
Brain tumor..............	0	0	2	2
Cerebrovascular disease.....	6	2	5	13
Totals...............	222 †	71 ‡	403	696

* The division of the patients into initial and residual groups of aphasia follows the suggestion of Luria discussed in an earlier chapter. The initial state corresponds to the six-month period immediately after injury. It is during this period that spontaneous recovery is said to occur. (See page 34.) The residual stage is that period beyond the sixth posttraumatic month when all or most spontaneous recovery is over. The language disabilities which exist at that time are usually permanent. For the purposes of this study only those patients who showed a *residual* aphasia were selected as subjects.
† Many of the individuals in this group continued to show aphasia disorders in their later course and were given a partial course of re-education. They were not used as subjects for the present study, since their defects were either minimal or limited to a single modality during the residual stage.
‡ It should be noted that seventy-one subjects showed a disorder of sufficient degree to be used in the present study. One of these patients died during the training period, and two others dropped out before training was completed, leaving a total of sixty-eight cases which were recorded in full.

Types of Aphasia Found. Table 4 shows the distribution of language disorders found in subjects of the study. The classification system follows the nomenclature established for the study as discussed in Chapter 4.

TABLE 4

DISTRIBUTION OF TYPES OF APHASIA OBSERVED IN THIS STUDY

Type	Frequency
Expressive-receptive........	17
Receptive.................	11
Expressive	30
Global...................	10
Total...............	68

Age Distribution of Subjects. The distribution of ages found among the subjects of the study at the time they began training are shown in Table 5.

TABLE 5

DISTRIBUTION OF SUBJECTS BY AGE

Type of Aphasia	Mean Age	Age Range
Expressive-receptive..........	24.1	19–34
Receptive.......	25.0	19–37
Expressive......	25.9	19–36
Global..........	29.5	23–38
	(Average) 25.8	(Over-all) 19–38

Vocational Backgrounds of Subjects.—Table 6 shows the distribution of vocational backgrounds found among the subjects. The work categories and the degrees of competence are taken from army records.

TABLE 6

VOCATIONS BEFORE ARMY SERVICE

Vocation	Competence	Type of Aphasia				
		E–R	R	E	G	Total
Salesman.........................	Skilled	1	0	1	2	4
Laborer, city......................	Skilled	7	3	12	4	26
Laborer, city......................	Unskilled	1	1	4	1	7
Laborer, farm.....................	Skilled	2	2	1	1	6
Laborer, farm.....................	Unskilled	6	3	2	0	11
Student..........................		0	2	7	1	10
Army............................		0	0	1	0	1
Unknown.........................		0	0	2	1	3
Total.........................						68

Legend for abbreviations used:
  E–R............Expressive-receptive
  R..............Receptive
  E..............Expressive
  G..............Global

Measuring the Effects of Training

Preinjury Educational Status.—The social service staff, by a search of the army records on each subject, supplemented in some cases by home visits, was able to secure the educational achievement status of each subject prior to his injury. This was accepted as a constant base for the pretraumatic educational level. The weaknesses of this as a true measure of educational ability are readily apparent.

Despite the accepted weaknesses, the data are considered to be of significant value for comparative purposes. The testing of the hypothesis that language loss can be recovered is not dependent in any way upon these data, yet their inclusion permits some evaluation in terms of the degree to which in an educational sense the subjects returned to their preinjury state.

The following table shows the distribution of preinjury educational achievement and the range of grades for the different types of aphasia seen in the study.

TABLE 7

PREINJURY EDUCATIONAL ACHIEVEMENT OF SUBJECTS

Type of Aphasia	Number	Mean Grade Level	Range of Grades
Expressive-receptive..............	17	9.4	3–12
Receptive.......................	11	9.5	2–12
Expressive......................	30	10.3	6–12
Global..........................	10	10.2	8–12
Total group..................	68	9.85	2–12

Two interesting facts are seen in Table 7. First, no subject had gone beyond high school before entering the army. Second, the mean of all the groups as well as the mean of each group was within

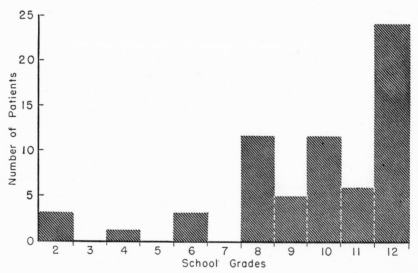

FIG. 2.—Educational achievement prior to injury as evidenced by highest school grade passed before entering army.

the high school level. Figure 2 shows graphically the prearmy educational achievement level of the subjects.

As the figure indicates, most of the subjects of the study had completed more than the eighth grade and fifty-one of the sixty-eight had either completed high school or were within the high school range at the end of their educational efforts prior to their injuries.

Achievement Test After Injury and Before Training.—Within the first two weeks after referral for training, the psychologist administered to each subject a progressive achievement test.[9] The elementary battery was used at this stage. A breakdown of the test performance permitted a separate score for reading, writing, spelling, and arithmetic. Training in these subjects was started on the level determined by the test.

Speech Performance.—During the first month of training, each teacher, psychologist, and social worker and the head of the Center, who had daily contact with the subjects, wrote descriptive paragraphs on their speech performance, noting the amount of verbalization, the use of sentences, the meaningfulness of verbal attempts, and the vocabulary used. From these paragraphs the writer later rated each subject on his speech performance.

Three psychologists, working independently, also used the paragraphs to rate the subjects. These independent ratings were made by individuals who at no time had contact with the subjects of the study. In all but four instances, perfect agreement was found on the four separate ratings. When disagreement was found at this stage, the highest rating given by any of the judges was used. This was done to offset any personal bias entering into the later judgment of improvement made in the speech performance area.

Table 8 shows the distribution of scores obtained on the pretraining administration of the educational achievement test. The scores are arranged in terms of the four types of aphasia.

This table shows that the subjects' mean postinjury educational level was within the early elementary grades. The highest accomplishment is seen in the expressive group, while the lowest is in the group with global aphasia. This is an entirely expected distribution in terms of the severity of the language function disability seen. Figure 3 shows the same distribution graphically expressed for the entire group.

---

[9] E. W. Tiegs and W. W. Clark, *Progressive Achievement Tests* (Hollywood, Calif.: California Test Bureau, 1943).

TABLE 8

PRETRAINING EDUCATIONAL ACHIEVEMENT OF SUBJECTS *

Type of Aphasia	Number	Mean Grade Level	Standard Deviation	Range of Grades
Expressive-receptive.......	17	3.5	1.0	2.1–4.8
Receptive...............	11	3.7	1.1	2.3–5.9
Expressive..............	30	4.1	1.3	2.9–6.6
Global.................	10	3.0	.8	2.2–4.2
Total group..........	68	3.7	1.2	2.1–6.6

* Ratings on speech performance are not included in this table, but will be shown later.

Figure 3 illustrates the grouping of the subjects in the early elementary grades. The mode is seen to fall at the third grade level, with sixty-one of the sixty-eight subjects at or below the fourth grade. It is also to be noted that none of the subjects was above the sixth grade in educational achievement prior to training.

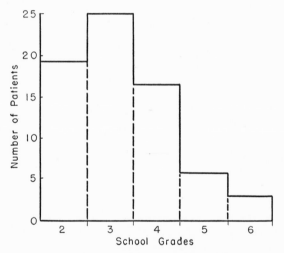

FIG. 3.—School grades prior to training as evidenced by scores on educational achievement tests.

Direct comparison of the total population before and after injury is shown in Table 9. From the data in this table it can be stated with confidence that there is a significant loss of educational ability in the language areas measured for these subjects. The correlation between the two sets of data indicates a slight tendency for the relative rank order of ability to remain the same. This is seen to be

TABLE 9

PRE- AND POSTINJURY EDUCATIONAL LEVELS

Statistical Measures Determined	Preinjury Grade Level	Postinjury Test Scores
Number....................	68	68
Mean grade..................	9.8	3.7
Standard deviation............	2.5	1.2

Statistical Interrelations Between the Pre- and Postinjury Educational Levels:

Mean grade difference............................	6.1
Standard error (mean grade difference).............	.3
t ratio...........................'...............	20.3
Level of significance (t tables)....................	Above 1%
Correlation coefficient............................	.36
Level of significance (r tables)....................	Above 1%

only a mild tendency, however, and the predictive value for any individual in the group would be low. This most probably means that no very accurate general prognostication concerning post-traumatic educational level can be made from a patient's preinjury educational history. In this study there were only two individuals who showed a shift opposite to the expected one; that is, they showed a higher educational ability by test score than the level at which they had left school. These subjects left school at the second grade level. Neither one had concluded his educational career, and both had failed to perform satisfactorily at the second grade level.

Summary of Pretraining Situation.—The data shown in the previous pages permit the following generalizations concerning the subjects before they began their re-education process:

1. Before trauma the subjects' educational levels extended from the second grade through the twelfth grade with the greatest number in the high school group.
2. After trauma, but before training, the subjects were all below the sixth grade level. The great majority were between the second and the fourth grade in educational achievement.
3. The order of educational achievement after trauma, for the four types of aphasia, starting at the top, was, as expected, expressive, receptive, expressive-receptive, and finally global.
4. The mean grade loss of the total group was about six grades. This was seen to be a significant loss.

5. There was noted a low positive correlation between the pretraumatic educational status and the postinjury educational
achievement level.

Re-education.—Following the pretraining testing period the
subjects were given formal training in four language areas, reading,
writing, spelling, and mathematics. In addition, speech training was
given whenever it was indicated. Speech was taught in two ways:
(*a*) At the beginning of the training process for some subjects,
work was done in developing recognition of verbal language symbols.
(*b*) Throughout the training process, speech correction was given
for errors of articulation and rhythm.

The teaching of these language areas by direct instruction was
supplemented by a planned extracurricular program. The additional
activities included occupational therapy, physiotherapy, and recreational therapy designed to alleviate the individual's paralysis; discussion groups, social experiences, field trips, and interward meetings
designed to assist the subjects in regaining some of their previous
social adjustments; and direct individual and group psychotherapy
designed to assist them in overcoming adjustmental problems that
they could not handle by themselves.

This over-all program was planned in accordance with the working principles developed at some length in earlier chapters. Each
subject's aphasia was considered as a defect affecting his total personality and as a limited speech problem.

The formal education was offered through the medium of teachers whose training and experience enabled them to effect changes in
the language areas efficiently. These teachers taught five days a
week. In addition to their contribution as instructors they were
instrumental in solving two difficult educational problems. The first
of these concerned instructional material, especially for the beginning period of training. No prepared material was available that
was suitable for the teaching of word substitutions or symbols. From
their earlier experiences with the preparation of workbooks for children they were able to prepare picture-word workbooks at an adult
level.[10]

The second area in which the teachers exhibited their unique
contribution was in the handling of motivation. As was pointed out
in Chapter 3, the aphasic adult has a number of personality deviations that make him a difficult student to teach. Among these many

---

[10] A master workbook based upon those used in this study is being prepared for
publication.

aberrations are such specific difficulties as lack of motivation, increased irritability, withdrawal and seclusiveness, reduced initiative, and a tendency toward catastrophic reaction to failure. The teachers' earlier experiences with children who showed different degrees of initiative and motivation prepared them to some degree for the task of motivating these adults. They were able to recognize the signs of the behavior abnormalities and offset them before they disrupted the classroom situations.

Recognizing the catastrophic reaction of the aphasic adult as a maximal display of the behavior shown by children when they were faced by frustration, the instructors were able to individualize training for the subjects to minimize the effects of frustration. In general, they were equipped to reduce the delays that would have been so common and so disrupting of a steady progression in learning.

Instructional material beyond the very beginning was also difficult to obtain. The subjects were unable to accept the use of the ordinary elementary texts. The situations were too infantile for their adult appreciation of the world. This lack of material was supplied for the most part by a series of texts obtained through the United States Armed Forces Institute. For writing instruction the need was met through Gardner's text on left-handed writing.[11] The teachers continued to face the problem of inadequate instructional material throughout the training program. In the later stages they adapted texts in widely separated areas for the language teaching purpose. In this way history, geography, and current events were the media through which language was taught.

The re-education program continued for approximately eighteen months. Classes met five days a week, six hours each day. The extracurricular work extended into the evenings and Saturdays. While furloughs were permitted, they were refused by the subjects during the first year of the Center's work. During the last six months a total of only fifteen furloughs were taken.

The following pages will show the results of this re-educational program.

Posttraining Data.—For the benefit of the staff, instructional conferences were held monthly or whenever the teachers indicated that a special problem needed discussion. At these conferences a discussion of progress, a review of successful and unsuccessful approaches, individual problems of the instructors and the subjects,

---

[11] Warren Gardner, *Left-handed Writing* (Danville, Ill.: Interstate Press, 1945).

and requests for evaluation were considered. Whenever the teachers indicated that a subject had plateaued in learning and seemed to have attained the maximum benefit of training, that subject was referred to the psychologist for examination.

Testing procedures at the conclusion of training included administration of tests to measure educational achievement level, intelligence, and, whenever indicated, personality characteristics. The educational achievement was again measured by the Progressive Achievement Test. Since in every instance a higher grade level of the test given at the beginning of training was used, it was not thought necessary to equate the forms. The results of this final test for educational achievement are seen in Table 10.

TABLE 10

FINAL LEVELS OF EDUCATIONAL ACHIEVEMENT

Type of Aphasia	Number	Mean Grade	Standard Deviation	Range of Grades
Expressive-receptive.......	17	8.7	2.2	5.2–11.6
Receptive...............	11	8.4	2.3	5.5–11.9
Expressive..............	30	9.9	1.6	7.1–11.8
Global.................	10	7.9	3.4	3.1–11.9
Total group..........	68	9.1	2.3	3.1–11.9

The data in this table support the following generalizations:

1. The expressive group attained the highest achievement, followed by the expressive-receptive, the receptive, and the global group.
2. The expressive group was most homogeneous of all the groups at the end of training. The global group is seen to cover almost the entire range of the elementary and high school grades.

Figure 4 indicates graphically the grade level of achievement for the group at the end of training.

As the figure indicates, the majority of subjects had reached the high school level at the conclusion of training. Forty-two of the sixty-eight subjects were at the secondary school level; only twenty-six were at the eighth grade or below. The mode of the distribution is seen to be at the eleventh grade.

Comparison of the Three Stages.—Table 11 compares the mean grade level of educational achievement at the three stages considered in this study: the preinjury educational status, the pretraining educa-

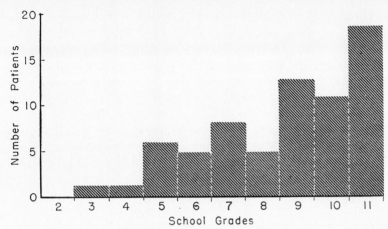

Fɪɢ. 4.—School grade levels after training as evidenced by scores on educational achievement tests.

TABLE 11

THREE STAGES OF EDUCATIONAL ACHIEVEMENT

Statistical Measures Determined	(1) Preinjury Status	(2) Pretraining Level	(3) Posttraining Level
Mean grade..............	9.8	3.8	9.1
Standard deviation........	2.5	1.2	2.3

Statistical Relationships Between the Three Stages

	Between (1) and (2)	Between (2) and (3)	Between (1) and (3)
Mean grade difference......	6.0	5.3	.7
Standard error of the difference.................	.3	.3	.3
t ratios.................	20.3	20.3	2.3
Level of significance (t tables)..............	Above 1%	Above 1%	1%
Correlation coefficients.....	.36	.31	.28
Level of confidence........	1%	1%	1%

tional achievement as measured by test, and the posttraining level measured by educational achievement test.[12]

---

[12] Table 11 includes only data on the four language areas, reading, writing, spelling, and mathematics. The data on speech performance will be presented in a later section.

The data presented in Table 11 permit the following generalizations:

1. The mean grade shows a return to approximately the same level after training as the subjects showed before their injury. The difference is seen to be only .7 of one grade. While this difference is shown to be statistically significant at a high level of confidence, for practical purposes it is a slight change.
2. The group is seen to have been more homogeneous before training than at either of the other periods.
3. There was a continuous tendency for the groups to maintain somewhat the same relative rank order at the three stages. This tendency is slight, however, and while it may serve to indicate that as a group the better educated show a higher pretraining level as well as a higher posttraining level, almost nothing could be said about the position that an individual member of the group might take.

Figure 5 expresses graphically the grade levels of the group at the same three stages of their development. It shows the extreme disparity between the postinjury, pretraining period and the other two periods. The graph shows the shift of the subjects in educational ability from the mode of the twelfth grade before injury, to

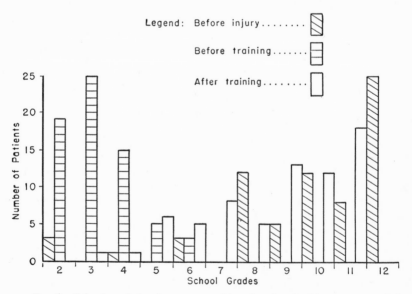

FIG. 5.—School grade levels as measured by educational achievement tests before and after training and by highest school grade passed before injury.

the third grade after injury, and back up to the eleventh grade after training.

Table 12 indicates that the greatest improvement and the highest level of attainment were made by the expressive group.[13] The

TABLE 12

EDUCATIONAL ACHIEVEMENT BY TYPE OF APHASIA

Type	Number	Pretraining		Posttraining		Mean Difference	Standard Error
		Grade	Standard Deviation	Mean Grade	Standard Deviation		
Expressive-receptive..	17	3.5	1.0	8.7	2.2	5.1	.25
Receptive...........	11	3.7	1.1	8.4	2.3	4.7	.27
Expressive...........	30	4.1	1.3	9.9	1.6	5.8	.20
Global.............	10	2.9	.8	7.9	3.4	5.0	.38

global group showed the lowest starting point and the lowest level of accomplishment, but their gain was greater than that made by the receptive group.

The expressive-receptive group started its training at the second lowest level and at the end was next to the highest in attainment. It also made the second greatest over-all gain. The receptive type began its training at a level just below the expressive group, and finished below both the expressive-receptive and the expressive groups. In terms of gain it made less improvement than any of the others.

The data also indicate that the global type, which was most homogeneous in terms of ability at the beginning of training, showed the greatest divergence after training. Some of the subjects in this group were at the very bottom of the total distribution, while others were almost at the top. The other groups showed an increase in spread of abilities but maintained approximately the same rank order that they had prior to training.

Table 13[14] shows the level of educational achievement for the total group in terms of four language areas, before and after training. The category of speech improvement, referred to earlier, is also included.

[13] E. Butfield and O. Zangwill, "Re-education in Aphasia," *Journal of Neurology, Neurosurgery and Psychiatry*, IX, New Series, No. 2 (April, 1946), 79.

[14] The data in Table 13 confirm the finding of Butfield and Zangwill's study. These authors say, "the most favorable outcome is obtained in those cases where symptoms are predominantly on the expressive side" (p. 79).

Table 13 shows that a significant change occurred during training in each of the categories. The order of improvement in the four language areas, taught formally, is seen to be (1) reading, (2) mathematics, (3) writing, and (4) spelling. A significant improvement is noted in the area of speech performance.

TABLE 13

BEFORE- AND AFTER-TRAINING LANGUAGE AND SPEECH LEVELS

Statistical Measures Determined	Reading Grade Levels	Writing Grade Levels	Spelling Grade Levels	Mathematics Grade Levels	Speech Perform-ance *
Before-training means..	3.2	3.9	4.0	3.8	1.8
Standard deviation.....	1.1	1.6	1.3	1.3	.8
After-training means...	8.4	9.2	9.3	9.1	3.9
Standard deviation.....	2.6	2.3	2.3	2.3	1.1
Mean difference.......	5.2	5.3	5.3	5.3	2.1
t ratios..............	17.85	18.82	19.38	18.08	16.21
Level of significance (t tables).............	1%	1%	1%	1%	1%
Correlation coefficients (differences).........	.30	.32	.34	.20	.29
Level of significance (r tables).............	1%	1%	1%	5%	5%

* Data based on rating scale described on page 53.

Figure 6 shows a distribution of gain made in terms of the four language areas and indicates the general tendency of the language areas to improve to almost the same degree. In part this was probably due to the stress that was placed upon the use of language *as it was recovered.* As soon as the students were found able to use language on a given conceptual level, all language practice material and exercises were designed to make use of that level. The greatest difficulty in this regard was noted in the area of mathematics, where as the graph indicates, some five students were unable to progress as much as one grade.

Butfield and Zangwill report that there was less improvement in the areas of reading, writing, and calculation than in the area of speech in their study.[15] Speech itself was not taught as a separate language area in the present study, but the improvement found in the area of speech performance was no greater than the improvement noted in other areas.

[15] *Op. cit.,* p. 78.

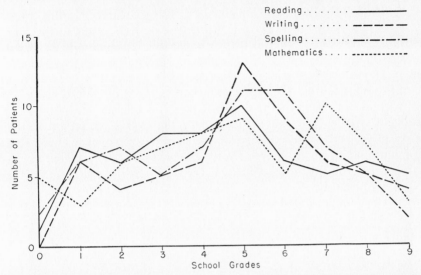

Fig. 6.—Number of school grades gained in reading, writing, spelling, and mathematics as measured by educational achievement tests given before and after training.

Recapitulation

On the preceding pages is indicated the general background of the subjects and of the present study; the selection of subjects for the study and the testing of the basic hypothesis of the study; the data that were collected to test whether or not patients who are aphasic as a consequence of cerebral insult are amenable to re-education. The pretraumatic levels of the subjects are shown in terms of their educational achievement. The assumption is made that an individual who has passed a particular grade in school prior to his injury can be said to have been *at least* on that grade level in the language areas in which we are interested. The mean grade level of educational achievement is seen to be 9.8 prior to injury. The mode of the distribution of pretraumatic educational level is seen to be at the twelfth grade, while sixty-one of the sixty-eight subjects had passed successfully at least eight grades of school.

Following their injuries the subjects are seen to be on a mean grade level of only 3.7, and their range of educational level was noted as being between the beginning of the second grade and the middle of the sixth grade. Of the four types of aphasia represented, the expressive group is at the highest level, followed by the receptive, the expressive-receptive, and finally the global type. The tendency of the groups to cluster about the means of their group, however, is seen to be in an exact reversal of this order. Forty-four of the subjects are noted as being at or below the third grade level, while the remaining twenty-two subjects range upward to the sixth grade.

The difference or loss of educational level as expressed in terms of grades is found to be approximately six. Loss of educational level by grades in terms of the different types of aphasia shows that the global type lost the most, followed by the expressive-receptive, the receptive, and finally the expressive type. The global group lost a significantly greater amount than the other three types, while the latter were grouped to the point that their losses, while different, were not significantly so.

The data presented indicating the improvement made as the result of training point to a gain of over five grades for the total group. This new level closely approximates the preinjury level of the group. In terms of the different types of aphasia and based upon pretraining levels, the greatest gain is shown by the expressive type, the next by the expressive-receptive type, followed by the global and then the receptive group. Improvement made in terms of the different language areas is seen to be approximately the same in each modality.

In speech performance, the one area not covered in the foregoing summary, an improvement was seen of two points on a five-point rating scale, with a total lack of speech at the bottom of the scale and normal or average speech expression at the top of the scale. It was seen that the total group showed a numerical improvement from 1.75 to 3.9. This was found to be a significant difference at an extremely high level of confidence.

One highly consistent factor, seen throughout the data so far presented, is the low positive correlation between the subjects' educational achievement rank order at the three stages. The tendency seemed to remain constant for the group to maintain to a slight degree their relative rank order in terms of language ability. Low positive correlation coefficients were found between (1) the pretraumatic and posttraumatic stages, (2) the pretraining and posttraining stages, and (3) even the preinjury and posttraining stages. The fact that the better educated students tended to remain at somewhat higher educational levels after injury and that the subjects who were highest in rank order of educational achievement after injury were also highest after training would indicate that, to the degree of significance that the statistics have, it would be possible to predict the amount of loss and amount of gain a particular individual would have were he to suffer a brain injury. It should be pointed out, however, that the actual correlations are so slight as to make this prediction hazardous at best.

Contributions from the Literature

Care of head-injured adults during the recent war has led to a number of publications concerned with training. This work has been largely in the hands of speech pathologists, and most of the published material has been in journals concerned with speech re-education. Sheehan [16] has said, "We have felt it worthwhile: some of the results are measurable enough, others show simply in the healthier and happier attitudes of those who leave us. We feel we can conclude that we have been able to hasten the process of re-education; that we have pushed it far beyond the level usually attained by the patient allowed to drift his own way without guidance." Anderson discussed in two papers a speech pathologist's working concept of aphasias, based upon eighteen cases studied over the past three years. She wrote that "he must discover whatever linguistic potential remains with the patient; he must evaluate this potential in terms of re-education in speech; he must plan to use this residuum most efficiently in speech therapy adapted to each individual." [17] The present writer would go beyond Anderson's statement and say that while the speech pathologist is succeeding in helping the patient regain his speech, the educator must be employed to assist the patient to recover all the language potentials that are only suggested by the speech specialist, while the clinical psychologist is needed to complete the patient's personality readjustment.

Peacher has made the only survey of speech disorders in World War II so far published. While this was a limited survey, it indicated the number of aphasic adults found in one general hospital. In this study Peacher found thirty-two patients showing dysphasia out of 120 patients exhibiting speech defects. Peacher speaks of rehabilitation and mentions that "definite improvement was noted in many instances following speech training." [18]

Backus, working at one of the army centers for the brain-injured, commented that "we are becoming increasingly optimistic as we work

---

[16] Vivian Sheehan, "Rehabilitation of Aphasias in an Army Hospital," *Journal of Speech Disorders*, XI (June, 1946), 153.

[17] Jeannette Anderson, *"Is* Is Not the Verb for Aphasia," *Journal of Speech Disorders*, XI (June, 1946), 137.

[18] W. G. Peacher, "Speech Disorders in World War II," *Journal of Speech Disorders*, X (June, 1945), 155–58.

with these patients and develop more effective techniques of rehabilitation." [19] It is unfortunate that no comparative figures are as yet available on the total number of aphasia patients re-educated during the war. Survey material was gathered by the Medical Department of the army but has not yet been released. Israel Wechsler expresses the viewpoint of many neurologists when he comments pessimistically on the possibilities of treatment: "It is very difficult to treat aphasia because the patient is so frequently inaccessible. Patient attempts at re-education by means of unimpaired senses—touch, vision, etc.— offer some hope." [20]

The studies mentioned serve to indicate the interest in the problem of re-education by speech pathologists, without offering more than discursive observations on the results achieved.

Butfield and Zangwill, however, did a statistical study of their patients, and the results they achieved in Great Britain make an interesting comparison with the results of the present study. [21] Using categories of improvement in which each subject was rated as either "Much Improved," "Improved," or "Unimproved," they found the following distribution: Much Improved—29; Improved—20; Unimproved—14. The determination of improvement was made by a rating scale based upon: "1. The senior member of the clinical staff's opinion. 2. The results of repeated psychometric testing. 3. The patient's work record in the speech therapy department." Butfield and Zangwill comment further that the ratings are in terms of relative improvement from the pretraining state. [22]

Using the Butfield and Zangwill rating scale on the subjects reported here would show the following distribution of improvement: Much Improved—35; Improved—25; Unimproved—8. These figures compare favorably, then, with the only other study indicating degree of improvement that is reported in the literature.

The literature was seen to be exceedingly meager on the subject of re-education and its effects. Several studies were reviewed that showed the viewpoint of students in the field to be in accord with the objective findings of this study. One study made in England, where statistical computations were made, was found to agree with the data offered in this study concerning the general effects of training, although some of the individual findings were not the same.

In general it can be concluded from the foregoing evidence that

---

[19] Ollis Backus, "Rehabilitation of Aphasic Veterans," *Journal of Speech Disorders*, X (June, 1945), 153–61.
[20] *Textbook of Clinical Neurology*, p. 334.
[21] *Op. cit.*, p. 75 ff.
[22] *Ibid.*, p. 77.

aphasia following brain injury is amenable to improvement. All the other studies reported used techniques of re-education in which the work was done entirely by speech pathologists, while in the present study the work of the speech pathologist was complemented by the work of instructors in each language modality. From this it can be inferred that the aphasic can be re-educated by a combination of teachers of speech and teachers of other language modalities. No comparative statistics are available at the present time to evaluate the two approaches.

Chapter 6

OTHER AREAS OF RESEARCH

As indicated earlier, several questions collateral to the basic one, the amenability of the aphasic patient to therapy, were considered important enough to be tested as by-products of the study. While not fundamental to the basic issue, data on these questions, it will be seen, are important to the therapist contemplating a program for aphasia training. It was seen by inspection that three such questions could be answered by the data, namely: (1) What is the most effective time to begin training the aphasic patient? (2) What is the relationship between measurable I.Q. and aphasia? and (3) What is the most effective way to use instructors in the training program?

The Most Effective Time to Begin Training

Butfield and Zangwill suggest that the results of training are improved if the re-education process begins as soon as possible after injury. In their study the group of aphasic patients who began their training before the end of the spontaneous recovery period showed the best results.[1] To offset the bias that would enter the data from results achieved on patients beginning during the spontaneous recovery period, only those subjects were selected whose training was started after the end of the sixth posttraumatic month. A preliminary survey of the subjects available for the study indicated that they fell roughly into two groups. One group started their training within the first posttraumatic year and the other group sometime after the end of the first posttraumatic year. Accepting this division of subjects, it was considered worth-while to test the hypothesis that training accomplishes more if started as soon as possible after the end of the first six months and before the end of the first year after injury than it does if training is delayed until after the end of the first posttraumatic year.

Data on Time to Begin Training. Table 14 shows the two groups in terms of the different types of aphasia in each group.

---

[1] E. Butfield and O. Zangwill, "Re-education in Aphasia," *Journal of Neurology, Neurosurgery and Psychiatry,* IX, New Series, No. 2 (April, 1946), 75–79.

The distribution of types is seen to be approximately the same in the two groups. While the number of expressive aphasias in the early group is greater than in the delayed group, there is also an increased number of the global type in the same group. Thus, very little bias in terms of types of aphasia is seen in the two groups.

TABLE 14

TYPES OF APHASIA SEEN IN EARLY AND DELAYED TRAINING GROUPS

Type	Group A (Training Begun During the First Year)	Group B (Training Begun After the First Year)	Totals
Expressive-receptive	9	8	17
Receptive	5	6	11
Expressive	16	14	30
Global	6	4	10
Totals	36	32	68

Table 15 shows the pre- and posttraining educational levels for the sixty-eight subjects, divided into two groups; the mean grade level of accomplishment before training and after training; the difference or gain made during training for each group; and the statistical relationship between the two groups. The means attained in the language areas, reading, writing, spelling, and mathematics are considered as the language level achieved. Speech performance is not considered, since it was not taught as a formal subject.

TABLE 15

COMPARISON OF RESULTS IN EARLY AND DELAYED GROUPS

Data Determined	Pretraining	Posttraining	Mean Difference	S.E.
Early Training—Number=36:				
Mean grade level	3.9	9.8	5.8	.16
Standard deviation	1.3	2.3	1.6	
Delayed Training—Number=32:				
Mean grade level	3.7	8.5	4.8	.15
Standard deviation	.7	1.7	2.3	

Intergroup Relationships:
Mean difference... 1.0
t ratio... 2.1
Level of significance (t tables)................................ 5%

Table 15 indicates that the two groups were equated within three tenths of a grade level at the beginning of training. The delayed group, which was slightly lower in mean ability, was more homogeneous. After training, the mean grade level is seen to be more than a grade better in the group whose training began within the first year. The delayed group continued to show a greater degree of homogeneity. The distribution of the differences between the pre- and posttraining stages, however, shows the gain made by the early group to be an average of almost one grade better than the gain made by the delayed group. This difference is seen to be significant in the sense that it would be expected to occur by chance in only five instances out of a hundred. A point of interest is seen in the deviation from the mean in the distribution of differences; the delayed group showed less homogeneity at this point than did the early group. The latter group showed a greater increase in ability, while the former spread improvement out much more.

Summary.—The data suggest that training started before the end of the first posttraumatic year results in greater achievement than does training that is started after the end of the first year.

I.Q. and Aphasia

The literature indicates that one of the problems concerning students in the field of the brain-injured adult is the part that intelligence plays in the after-injury state of the patients. Freeman and Watts report that, at the time when Fritsch and Hitzig did their original work on the electrical excitation of the brain in 1870, the "argument in regard to the intellectual functions and their relationship to the frontal region became even more complicated, and at times acrimonious, as new bits of evidence pro and con became assembled, and . . . that the argument is in process of development even at the present time."[2] In the more limited field of aphasia, this argument is just as far from a solution today.

Weisenberg summarized the opinions of many investigators when he said, "The extent to which intelligence may be said to be affected is a moot point. Some investigators have held that intelligence suffers because speech is disturbed while others have held that speech is disturbed because of the intellectual disorder."[3]

---

[2] W. Freeman and J. W. Watts, *Psychosurgery* (Springfield, Ill.: Charles C. Thomas, Publisher, 1942), p. 21.

[3] T. Weisenberg and K. McBride, *Aphasia* (New York: The Commonwealth Fund, Division of Publications, 1935), p. 70.

Marie believed that true aphasia was invariably distinguished by the presence of a general intellectual defect and a special defect of language.[4] Head was of the opinion that "all these processes which suffer in Aphasia are essentially psychical and, in so far as they are defective, the capacity of the mind is restricted." [5]

Jackson concluded that because ". . . the speechless man has thought as far as reviving images go . . . he can still think, can still have certain relations of likeness and unlikeness. He can bring two images into coexistence—existence in one unit of time—but cannot, without speech, organize the connection." [6]

Kennedy and Wolf say that ". . . there is a distinction between intellectual defect and aphasia, thought is possible without words and defective speech can exist as something apart from intelligence, ideation, attention, memory, and the power of association." [7]

A summary of the opinion expressed leads to the belief that the aphasia patient has an intellectual defect, either as the result of his aphasia or as a separate entity. To show the relationship between measurable I.Q. and aphasia, the following data were collected during preparation of the present study:

1. The pretraumatic I.Q. of each subject, obtained from the Army General Classification Test
2. The before-training I.Q., obtained from individual administration of the Wechsler-Bellevue scales performance section [8]
3. The after-training I.Q., obtained from a final administration of the total Wechsler-Bellevue scale

Table 16 indicates the distribution of mean I.Q.'s at the three stages and the interrelationships between the mean scores obtained.

In their pretraumatic state the subjects were well within the accepted normal I.Q. range (90–110) in ability. The standard deviation of their mean scores shows that they tended to cluster about the mean in an expected manner for an unselected group from the general population. The lower mean intelligence test score indicated in the second column shows the loss of efficiency in mental function that

---

[4] Pierre Marie, cited in F. Moutier, *L'Aphasie de Broca* (Paris: G. Steinhil, 1908), p. 375 ff.

[5] Henry Head, *Aphasia and Kindred Disorders of Speech* (New York: The Macmillan Co., 1926), p. 211.

[6] J. H. Jackson, cited in "Hughlings Jackson on Aphasia," edited by Henry Head, *Brain*, XXXVIII (1915), p. 14.

[7] F. Kennedy and A. Wolf, "The Relation of Intellect to Speech Defect in Aphasia Patients," *Journal of Nervous and Mental Diseases*, LXXXIV (August, 1936), 125–26.

[8] David Wechsler, *Measurement of Adult Intelligence* (Baltimore: The Williams & Wilkins Co., 1944).

is expected after a head injury. At this stage, the group showed less variability in test scores. The third mean I.Q. level indicates a tendency on the part of the total group to approach their pretraumatic abilities after training. Not only do they approximate their earlier test scores, but the distributions show about the same dispersion.

In the second part of the table, the three columns indicate the loss of ability on mental tests, the gain through general language improve-

TABLE 16

I.Q. AT THREE STAGES

Statistical Measures Determined	(1) Pretraumatic	(2) Posttraumatic	(3) Posttraining
Mean I. Q...................	98.5	70.4	92.1
Standard deviation...............	13.6	9.0	12.2

Interstage Relationships

	(1) and (2)	(2) and (3)	(1) and (3)
Mean difference................	28.1	21.7	6.4
Standard error.................	1.6	1.3	2.0
t ratio.......................	18.5	16.3	3.1
Level of significance (t table)........	Above 1%	Above 1%	1%
Correlation coefficients............	.39	.50	.46
Level of significance (r table)........	1%	1%	1%

ment, and the apparent permanent loss. All the data collected indicate that the figures showing loss and gain are significant and are not due to chance.

The correlation between the first two stages indicates a tendency for the subjects with the highest intellectual ability, as measured by intelligence tests, to show higher ability after their injuries. To an even greater degree, the subjects who were high in their pretraining ability were also highest in their posttraining ability at test performance.[9] The rank order of ability in terms of the pretraumatic state is seen to be somewhat the same after training. An inference may be that the educator can predict posttraining scores from posttraumatic scores with some degree of confidence.

---

[9] While part of this higher correlation may be explained by the fact that the same test was used for before- and after-training I.Q.'s, the fact that memory loss is one of the most common signs of brain injury tends to offset the practice effect.

I.Q. for Different Types of Aphasia.—Table 17 shows the mean I.Q. change at the same three stages for the different types of aphasia.

Column 3 in this table shows that the highest mean I.Q. before injury was obtained by the global type, followed by the expressive, the expressive-receptive, and receptive groups in order. The distributions of each group are seen to be as expected for unselected groups.

TABLE 17

MEAN I.Q. LEVELS FOR DIFFERENT TYPES OF APHASIA
AT THREE STAGES

Type (1)	No. (2)	Pretraumatic		Pretraining		Posttraining	
		Mean I.Q. (3)	S.D. (4)	Mean I.Q. (5)	S.D. (6)	Mean I.Q. (7)	S.D. (8)
Expressive-receptive....	17	93.6	13.5	67.2	7.0	88.1	9.6
Receptive..............	11	93.5	17.3	69.3	6.9	88.7	13.1
Expressive............	30	100.8	12.7	73.7	10.3	93.3	18.4
Global...............	10	105.3	7.6	67.0	7.3	89.6	17.4

Column 5 indicates, however, that after injury the group with the highest mean score was the expressive, followed by the receptive, the expressive-receptive, and finally the global type. Column 7 shows that the highest final level was achieved by the expressive group and the next highest by the global, followed by the receptive and expressive-receptive groups. The order expressed here indicates that pretraumatic abilities may account in some degree for the final level achieved for the global group. The most seriously affected group in language, the global aphasias, showed a higher mean level than did the receptive and the expressive-receptive groups. The latter showed less disability in the pretraining state. Differences between the final I.Q. levels achieved for the last three groups are seen to be insignificant.

The expressive group showed a much greater tendency to scatter in their final scores, while the expressive-receptive group was certainly the most homogeneous at the conclusion of training.

Distribution Over the Group.—Figure 7 expresses graphically the distribution of mean I.Q. levels for the total group. It shows the dissimilarity between the I.Q. distribution of the subjects at the pretraining stage and at the other two stages, before injury and after injury.

The graph also indicates the approximate similarity between the preinjury and the posttraining distributions.

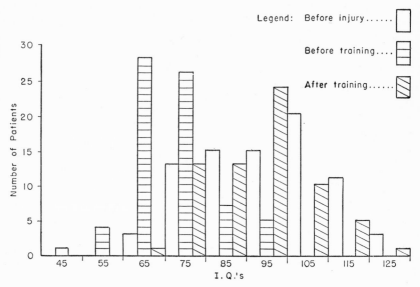

Fig. 7.—Distribution of I.Q.'s obtained by psychological tests before injury and before and after training.

The data presented here appear to bear a close relation to the data given in Chapter 5 on changes in educational level. This relation can best be expressed in the following correlations between I.Q. changes and educational changes:

1. Correlation between loss of educational achievement and loss of I.Q. after injury . . . . + .63

2. Correlation between gain in educational achievement and gain in I.Q. during training . . . . + .69

3. Correlation between preinjury, posttraining educational level differences and preinjury, posttraining I.Q. differences . . . . + .64

These data indicate that there is a considerable relationship between the aphasic adult's I.Q. and his educational achievement as shown by test scores.

Summary.—The foregoing data indicate that the aphasic adult tends to make lower scores on standard intelligence tests after his injury than he did before it. They also show that, with recovery of his language processes, the aphasia patient tends to show a recovery of ability on intelligence tests that approximates his pretraumatic ability. This leads to the conclusion that there is some predictive value in pretraumatic intelligence test scores. The high correlations seen between educational gains and losses at the three stages of the study indicate that I.Q. and education are very probably one and the same when they are measured by test in the aphasic adult. The data generally indicate that, while there is a measurable loss of I.Q. after injury, this loss is frequently not permanent and may be reversed through training.

Use of Instructors

Using some of the data shown in Chapter 5, information was obtained on the most effective use of teachers in the re-education program. It was believed by the writer that a single teacher for all academic instruction could accomplish more than different teachers used for each area to be taught. To test this belief the following data were collected.

The subjects were divided into two groups: Group *A,* where all instruction was offered by a single teacher for all material, and Group *B,* where different teachers were used for each course of instruction. Selection for the groups was made on a random basis, namely, the order in which the patient was accepted for training in the Center. To equate the groups for the different types of aphasia, the last twelve patients reported to the Center were assigned to groups on the basis of diagnosis. It was found to be impracticable to continue separate grouping for fourteen of the subjects because of problems of administration beyond the control of the writer. This was mainly due to the fact that these subjects were moved to distant wards during training, for surgery or other medical treatment. This made it impracticable to teach them through the single teacher method exclusively. They were not used in compilation of the data shown later. This left twenty-seven subjects in each group.

Table 18 shows the distribution of the two groups in terms of type of aphasia. There was approximately an equal number of each type represented in the two groups.

Table 19 shows the mean grade level for subjects in the two groups at the pretraining and posttraining stages, the difference or

TABLE 18

TYPES OF APHASIA IN DIFFERENT TEACHING GROUPS

Type	Group A, Taught by Single Instructor	Group B, Taught by Many Instructors	Totals
Expressive-receptive........	4	5	9
Receptive................	5	6	11
Expressive...............	15	11	26
Global..................	3	5	8
Totals..............	27	27	54

gain that each group made, and the significance of the difference between the two groups.

Table 19 indicates that the two groups were well equated in terms of pretraining mean grade levels. After training it is noted that only a two-tenths mean grade difference appears in the attain-

TABLE 19

COMPARISON OF SINGLE TEACHER AND MULTIPLE TEACHER METHODS

Statistical Measures Determined	Pretraining	Posttraining	Difference	S.E.
Group A, Single Instructor (Number=27):				
Mean grade levels............	3.7	9.3	5.6	.21
Standard deviations...........	1.2	2.0	1.9	
Group B, Multiple Instructor (Number=27):				
Mean grade levels.............	3.7	9.5	5.8	.22
Standard deviations...........	1.0	2.1	2.0	

Intergroup Relationships:
Mean difference (grade levels)..................................... .2
t ratio of mean differences....................................... .06
Level of significance.................................. Not significant

ment of the two groups. Statistically, this difference is seen to be below significance. These data suggest that there was little if any difference between the results achieved by the two methods used.

Objective Results

The results achieved with sixty-eight aphasic adults in an eighteen-month re-education program showed objectively that the language problem involved can be materially reduced. The data collected indicated that the following direct changes took place in the subjects during the training period:

1. (Prestudy estimate.) Loss of approximately six school grades between mean educational status before and after injury
2. Mean gain of slightly better than five school grades between pre- and post-training educational achievement levels
3. Slight, although significant, mean loss of educational achievement between before-injury and after-training periods
4. Slight, but significant, tendency for rank order of subjects to remain the same throughout the three stages studied
5. In terms of different types of aphasia, highest level attained after training in expressive group, followed in order by expressive-receptive, receptive, and global groups
6. In terms of improvement in language area, the order is slightly different; greatest gain by expressive group, followed by expressive-receptive, global, and finally receptive groups
7. In terms of speech improvement (treated separately throughout study), change amounting to over two steps on a five-point scale (The scale used extended from total lack of speech at one end to normal speech at the other.)
8. In terms of other formal language areas taught, greatest gain made in reading, followed by mathematics, writing, and spelling in that order (The improvement made in these areas was seen to be consistent for the entire group. A marked tendency was seen for the four areas to improve together.)

Data were also collected during the study that concerned the relationship between aphasia and the intellectual functioning ability of the subjects. The literature in this area was reviewed, and a considerable difference of opinion was noted among authorities. One group held that intellectual ability is always affected in aphasia and that this defect is separate from the language problem. Another group believed that the language defect and the intellectual ability of the individual aphasic adult were one and the same thing. This study offers no definite solution to the problem. The data, however, indicate that in terms of the subjects' abilities as measured by standard intelligence tests the following inferences can be drawn:

1. Marked decline in I.Q. after injury
2. Almost equal increase in I.Q. after training
3. High degree of correlation between gains made in language function and in I.Q.

The writer does not intend to argue that intelligence and the results of intelligence tests are the same, but reports only that these changes were seen to occur. However, to the degree that the intelligence tests used to measure the I.Q. in the present study did measure intellectual functioning ability, it can be said with some confidence that the intellectual and language problems were the same.

The data substantiated the hypothesis that early training culminates in greater success than training which starts after the end of the first posttraumatic year. In the two groups compared in the present study, an increased improvement was noted in those who started within the first year. Their mean attainment level was also noted as being higher at the conclusion of the training program.

Finally, the findings indicate that teachers can be used in either of two ways and the results achieved will be approximately the same. In the study, one group was taught by a single teacher for all its formal language training, the other group had different teachers for each language area. The results indicate no significant difference in the accomplishment of the two groups.

Implications of Research Findings

Use of Schoolteachers as Instructors.—One of the most important observations that can be made from the study reported concerns the use of experienced elementary-school teachers as instructors in the formal language areas of the program. While it does not seem radical to use elementary-school teachers as instructors in reading, writing, spelling, and arithmetic, to the best of the writer's knowledge it had never previously been attempted. Those studies which report the type of instruction used refer to speech pathologists as the sole members of the instructional staff. In the one study in the literature that does report objective findings, it was mentioned that the re-education was in the hands of a speech pathologist. It has already been indicated that the results obtained in that study showed a wide differential between the improvement noted in the different language areas. In the present study, however, all the language areas were seen to improve to approximately the same degree. It is felt that this was due in large part to the use of experienced teachers as instructors in each formal language area.

The teachers brought to the program educational techniques that were easily adaptable to the levels of the aphasic subjects. Their knowledge and use of instructional material at the elementary levels of learning appeared to facilitate considerably the learning process.

Their experience and skill in motivating children at the early stages of learning made the extremely difficult task of motivating the aphasic adults considerably easier. In retrospect it seems obvious that teachers, through their training and education, would possess skills and knowledge of teaching that speech pathologists would not be expected to have. The division of work in the present study between the teachers of the formal language areas and the teachers of speech freed both groups for the part of the total problem for which they were best qualified. On the basis of the results achieved in this study, it can be said that future programs for the re-education of aphasic adults should utilize the services of both elementary-school teachers and speech pathologists, working in collaboration.

Checking Educational Levels.—Another direct inference from the data presented is the use that can be made of information concerning the aphasic adult's educational and intellectual levels before and after injury. With some confidence, based upon these data, future training for aphasic adults can be undertaken with the knowledge that more successful resolution of the language problem can be expected when the I.Q. level at the preinjury state is found to be high. If this information is not available, similar, although not as accurate, prognostication of success can be made from the preinjury educational achievement level of the individual. The type of aphasia that the individual aphasic adult exhibits is also of considerable value in prognosticating the degree of recovery, since the study shows that the various types tend to improve in different degrees.

Use of a Total Program.—The results of the present study also indicate that there was merit in the effort made in planning the program so that the nonlanguage personality abnormalities of the subjects would be obviated. The fact that, of the sixty-eight subjects re-educated and rehabilitated, all but six were able to take their places in society in a useful capacity points to the advantages accruing from a total program. As in any program of education, the problems of rapport, motivation, and morale were considered as very important. Recognizing the effect that brain injury frequently has upon the individual and providing individual and group psychotherapy and social, occupational, and recreational activities, in addition to the formal program, contributed substantially, it is felt, to the rehabilitation secured. An inference that can be drawn from this appears to be that the aphasic adult needs more than formal re-education in skill functions; he needs a total rehabilitation. From this, the writer believes, future educational programs can expect that maximal results will be obtained only when the breadth of the problem is recognized and the curriculum includes an opportunity for the aphasic adult to overcome his maladjustments with the assistance of competent professional personnel.

The study suggests several other areas worthy of theoretical consideration. One of these relates to the manner in which the aphasic subjects appeared to regain their language facilities. An example of the process at one stage of learning will serve as an illustration.

Method of Retraining.—At the beginning of training it was necessary for each aphasic subject, regardless of the type of his aphasia, to learn to substitute words as symbols for objects or animals. Many lesson periods were spent in each language area using different stimuli before the first such substitute association was made. For example, the first word substitute used in a particular case was the word *man*. Pictures of men were shown in different situations; the word man was printed on the blackboard and copied by the patient; the phonetic elements involved were taught; a figure of a man was modeled in clay by the instructor and then by the patient; during this process the instructor would repeat the word man at intervals and ask the patient to imitate the pronunciation of the word. The printed word man was constantly before the patient on the blackboard. It was found that the repetition of the word by the teachers, whenever the topic was under discussion, and the simultaneous appeal to the other sense modalities while the word was being repeated, led to an eventual association of the word with the stimuli. This process frequently went on for several weeks before the subject would gain the desired Gestalt. After the word man was recognized and could be repeated meaningfully by the subject on the first presentation of a stimulus, a second word substitute would be started, for example, the word *dog*. It was observed that, as soon as a short series of such Gestalts was obtained—the series rarely going above five and frequently as few as three—the subject would be able to recognize any single naming word used. Further word-building was found to be unnecessary. New words were added over a comparatively short time by simple exposure of a stimulus. It was inferred from this that the learning process for the aphasic adult was one of gaining a Gestalt at a particular level. Once that Gestalt had been obtained and somewhat fortified, the subject could recall from his preinjury vocabulary without needing to relearn a new vocabulary or without needing to appeal to other sense modalities.

The foregoing illustration of one phase of relearning suggests that training programs for aphasia disorders should be planned on the basis of stimulating a series of progressively more difficult Gestalts rather than a program which builds up a wide experience level at each stage of learning. From this, a study planned to measure the learning process in aphasic adults as compared with the method of learning of approximately the same material by children in the elementary school seems feasible.

Function of the Dominant Hemisphere.—Another implication from the study is one concerning the function of the so-called dominant hemisphere (see pages 28 ff.). It is suggested by the data gathered for the present study as well as by a review of the literature that only the left cerebral hemisphere in all people is concerned with language on the symbolic level—in other words, that speech and language may be the function of the left hemisphere of the cortex only. If this is true, then the re-education process effects a reintegration of the cerebral function in the left hemisphere when it is successful, and it fails to succeed, in certain instances, because of the destruction of too much cortical tissue in the left hemisphere, the remaining tissue in that hemisphere being insufficient to produce the integration necessary. A thorough study of the literature in this area, a careful study of aphasic patients following localized removal of tissue from the left hemisphere, and a study of the effects of localized damage to the right hemisphere should throw some interesting light upon the manner in which the cerebral cortex is organized in terms of cerebral dominance. Such a study might also assist in making more successful prognostications of the recovery of future aphasic patients.

Possibility of Rehabilitation.—A final inference can be drawn from observations made on the subjects of the study. Throughout the training program it was seen that there was a constant and marked degree of change in their nonlanguage behavior characteristics. As they regained their language facility and obtained insight into their behavior, they tended more and more toward the patterns of the noninjured. This leads to the implication that previous studies which have reported so many permanent behavioral abnormalities in brain-injured patients were observing only a limited portion of behavior, at a particular time in the recovery process, and were considering these personality characteristics as permanent. While no generalizations can be drawn from a small study of the present type that would apply to all brain-injured adults, it can be said that the training program used in this study succeeded in obviating many common personality aberrations in the aphasic subject. To the extent that these problems exist as a result of the brain injury itself, and not the aphasia, training and psychotherapy should be able to overcome them in many brain-injured adults. This also suggests that future observations and research in the personality of brain-injured patients should consider the changing nature of the disorder, especially when psychotherapy is being used to assist in rehabilitation.

PART III

APHASIA THERAPY AND THERAPISTS

Chapter 7

THEORY AND WORKING PRINCIPLES

To this point the present volume has presented two phases of the complex disorder known as aphasia. Part I has shown the research findings that underlie the present study. An analysis has been made of the literature dealing with the etiology of aphasia, the classification of the many types of aphasia, and the commonly seen and verifiable nonlanguage behavior characteristics of the brain-injured patient. Part II has dealt with the collection of data bearing on several important but previously unverified questions concerning aphasia and its resolution. In this latter section it has been shown objectively that the aphasic patient can be re-educated and rehabilitated. The data also permitted analysis that bore upon such important aspects of the training process as the most effective time to begin re-education, the relationship between measurable I.Q. and aphasic disabilities, and some of the methods for using instructors in the training program. Part III will deal with the theory and working principles of aphasia therapy and will give some practical suggestions for re-education of aphasic adults. These latter have grown out of the program here reported, in which some seventy aphasic individuals were rehabilitated, and the writer's experiences with aphasic patients since the recent war.

Working Theory from the Literature

Aphasia as a Disorder of the Total Reaction Pattern.—Growing out of the writer's experience with the recovery of aphasic patients and out of the comparatively large literature on the etiology of aphasia came the basic concept of the disorder upon which his program of rehabilitation is founded. Differing rather sharply from previously held theories that aphasia is a disorder of speech or a language problem, narrowly conceived, it is held here that aphasia is a disorder affecting the patient's *total reaction pattern* due to a disturbance of the integrating capacity of the cortex. This working theory stresses the necessity for considering the patient as an individual in need of re-establishing the use of neural capacities which

85

are present and potentially functional, but which are blocked from use by the pathological condition existing within the cortex.

Arising from this concept is the need for developing an all encompassing rehabilitation program which deals with every facet of the individual and his personality, both physical and psychological. It demands thorough evaluation of pre- and postmorbid behavior as well as constant vigilance to adapt the training process to the needs of the individual rather than to any preconceived therapist-based concept of a common disorder. Primarily, the concept of the holistic effect of the brain injury upon the individual leads to the treatment of the individual rather than the treatment of the disorder.

Use of Nomenclature in Planning Therapy.—Review of the conflicting systems of nomenclature leads to the development of an operational classification system which embodies a few generally accepted indices. For the purpose of planning and implementing therapy, it is seen that four useful categories encompass all the patients and permit the development of useful therapeutic generalizations. In consequence the four-part system discussed in Chapter 4 was devised. The division of the patients into these four categories, Global, Expressive-receptive, Receptive, and Expressive, is based upon the need for a satisfactory point for considering the beginning steps in therapy. While the plan takes cognizance of the generally accepted motor and sensory facets of the problem, it also permits a separate categorization for the complex noncommunicating patients whose disorders are so severe that separate motor or sensory elements could not be parceled out. The classification system suggested is not meant to be anything more than a rough approximation of the general categories into which the patients may fall for the beginning of training. Thus, the global patients after making their first steps in recovery are rediagnosed and listed in one of the other categories. Likewise, many of the mixed expressive-receptive patients are reclassified as one or the other of their presenting problems becomes obviated. The only purpose for the original classification is held to be the focus for the onset of re-education. With this purpose in mind the classification proposed is held to be of considerable value to the therapist.

Recognition of Behavioral Signs.—The third major working principle derived from the literature and based upon the writer's experience is the need for considering at every stage of rehabilitation the common behavioral manifestations that set the cortically injured patient apart from the rest of the population. These observed behavioral mannerisms led to development of the widespread approach used in the reported study and found so useful that it is advocated for all aphasia therapy. In the training program discussed in Chapters 5 and 6 these verifiable modes of behavior led to many procedures not widely discussed in the literature in relation to re-education. First, they led to the author's conviction that there is a definite place for a psychological approach to the aphasia problem in the rehabilitation program. Certainly it is held that, whoever the therapist might be, there is need for a thorough grounding in the psychological performance of the individual suffering from aphasia if therapy is to be maximally beneficial. Second, they led to the need for developing an intensive orientation to the psychology of the brain-injured adult for everyone concerned in the resolution of his problem. Third, it is easily seen from a study of the reported behavioral manifestations what an important part their recognition plays in the planning of the therapeutic program. To illustrate this latter point, the recognition of increased fatigability in the brain-injured adult leads to curriculum planning that includes short lesson and therapeutic sessions intermingled with frequent rest periods, especially during the early stages of training. The recognized loss of initiative on the part of the patient leads to a greater need for developing stimulation and motivation than would be true otherwise. In like manner each of the discussed behavioral signs leads to preplanning to offset their possible deleterious effect upon recovery. Finally, the recognition of these factors and the vital part they play in the patient's own self-concept and ego development led to the concept discussed previously, which bears repetition because of its importance, namely, that therapy must be aimed at the *individual* and not at the disorder.

Principles Developed from the Re-education Process

The Aphasic Patient as an Individual.—The opportunity to work through the problems of aphasic adults reported in an earlier section brings one to the formation of a series of additional useful concepts for the therapist planning to work in the field of aphasia therapy. The first of these is the concept of the aphasic adult as an individual possessing a particular personality because of his biological determination, his early environmental conditioning, and the effects of his brain injury. This latter addition to the usual concept of the developing personality of the individual in our society consists of the effect of the brain pathology itself with its consequent realignment of neural potential and function; the increased inability to inhibit basic personality drives; the enforced alteration of self-concepts and ego development; and the forces inherent in the physical convalescence as well as the altered physical condition. It also seems more and more apparent that the patients reported on did not develop a so-called "organic personality," but rather seemed to possess and to project the same basic personalities that they had in their premorbid condition. The major sign of change was not in their personality type but in the manner in which it was projected. Whereas they had previously been able to sublimate direct action through the medium of language in one of its forms, following their traumatic experience they found themselves frequently unable to communicate in any satisfactory way or manner. This deprivation of a satisfactory avenue for the expression of their internal needs, added to their actual physiological loss of inhibitory control over voluntary action, made them appear to be new and different persons. Close observation over long periods of time revealed, however, that basically they were unchanged. Their internal drives and needs were unaltered, and only their method of relating these internal forces to the world was different. (In this connection see Halstead's discussion on the P factor in his recent volume on the activity and function of the frontal lobes.[1])

Withdrawal in the Aphasic Patient.—Having previously been able to communicate with their environment, aphasic patients find themselves isolated by an inability to communicate. This causes what has previously been described as their seclusiveness and withdrawal. When these characteristics are seen in brain-injured patients, it is usually true that the patients possessed these same traits in their premorbid condition. Outgoing individuals, on the other hand, often become more outgoing after injury. Some patients become isolated, not because of an internal drive in that direction, but because of an inability to relate to a communicating world with which they cannot communicate. Previously able to control their behavior voluntarily, they frequently find themselves to be lacking in inhibition of their impulses. This lack of internal control and a recognition of its impact upon their society tends to increase their desire to withdraw. Aphasic patients show that their lack of intellectual integration, leading to a decrease in their ability to project real meaning into their behavior, tends to make them easy prey to their innermost conflicts. Thus, those patients whose basic drives tend to make them

---

[1] Ward C. Halstead, *Brain and Intelligence* (Chicago: University of Chicago Press, 1947), p. 84 ff.

introversive in their behavior become more and more withdrawn, while the outgoing patients tend more and more to act out their hostilities, to reject society, and to fail to appreciate social approval or disapproval. From these observations it becomes apparent that what is seen in the behavior patterns of aphasic patients is an extension of their premorbid personalities rather than any single "organic" mold into which they all fall because of the coincidence of brain injury among them.

Re-education of the Whole Person.—The effect of this concept upon therapy should easily be seen. Re-education as well as total rehabilitation can be planned only upon an individual basis. This is especially true in the early stages of training. It is necessary to plan for a therapeutic program that will meet the individual needs of the patient rather than to plan to reduce a language disability through a direct training or educative program only. This concept also introduces the necessity for including planned psychotherapy in every aphasic adult's program. It is to be noted that a considerable portion of the aphasic patient's behavior is not directly caused by the physiological fact of the brain injury, but rather by the patient's new concept of self. The working principle derived from this insight is that the total therapeutic program (psychological, physical, educational, and speech) must consider the whole person; that the aphasic adult must be considered as a thinking, talking, acting individual whose level of performance is set by the limits of his physiological and intellectual capacity. Whatever behavior he presents must be considered as maximal behavior for him at that time in terms of his needs, his desires, and his abilities.

From this concept, too, it is believed to follow that the previously held concept of the aphasic adult as being the same person he was prior to his injury, or as having the potentiality of becoming the same person again through training and rehabilitation, must be discarded. The aphasic adult, even after maximal return of function and re-established personality, must be looked upon as a new individual possessing the same inherited constitutional factors and the same early conditioning background, but different cortical capacity, new cortical integrative patterns, and a new concept of self. The goals of therapy must be in terms of this new individual, of his potential, of his new energy level. If these new factors are not and cannot be recognized by the patient, assistance in developing a recognition of them must be an integral part of the therapeutic program.

Goals

The mention of goals in the preceding paragraph introduces a very important factor that must be considered in aphasia training. It became evident in the re-education program reported that goal seeking and goal recognition played an important part in the eventual success obtained. It was seen and has become a standard working principle of the writer that both the therapist and the patient must recognize, accept, and work toward a worth-while and achievable goal. Goal seeking and goal recognition are conceived in two parts. First, there must be an acceptance of the long-term, eventual goal. While in the early stages of recovery this may be a vague and seemingly unattainable goal far in the distant future, it must be restated and re-evaluated at many stages thereafter. As progress is noted and the patient begins to gain new insights and new concepts of self, the future and eventual goal should become more real, more practical, and more attainable. Secondly, recovery must be directed in terms of the immediate, almost day-by-day goals. The achievement of these short-term goals must be constantly related to the final goal. The patient must be constantly aware of the direction of his striving, the success he is having, and the need for continuous effort. This more than any other single factor seems to increase motivation. Generally speaking, it is found that the goals must be eminently practical and realistic.

An illustration of the effect of goal recognition and goal activity may be seen in one patient who, despite his extreme language handicap, maintained his premorbid goals intact. By vocation a salesman, his particular occupation required rapid, clear speech, split-second decisions, and rapid translation from abstract material into a concrete numerical symbolism. It was clearly seen in the light of this patient's disability that the goal of returning to this vocation at the level previously occupied was completely unrealistic at that time. At best that previous goal was far beyond any hopes of being obtained in a comparatively short year or two of training and most probably would never again be a worth-while goal for this patient. In consequence it was necessary to work through the patient's problem with him, to give him a more realistic understanding of himself, and to give him an understanding of what might be expected from training. Through psychotherapy a new and more real goal gained some acceptance.

This same patient illustrated the need for relating the daily language retraining to the final goal. Until the patient was able to perceive the relationship between what he was doing each day and his final achievement, progress was almost nonexistent. He appeared to be unable to summon a sufficient degree of energy to retain any of the material that was presented and apparently learned each day. As he gained insight into the process of re-education, as his total goals were worked through and became acceptable to him, and as he was able to see the day-by-day goals, his motivation increased. External stimulation was less necessary as his ego needs were perceived and were met, and learning and growth proceeded at an accelerated pace.

The problem of goals involves another interesting process met with in aphasia therapy that is largely different from other therapeutic problems. By the very nature of the aphasic adult's problem he appears to have lost most of his initiative. His planning capacity is impaired, he almost invariably shows signs of impaired concentration, and frequently he is unable to use good practical judgment. (These factors are discussed at some length in Chapter 3.) Upon the recognition of these personality deviations in any particular patient, it is found to be necessary to develop goals for the patient, working through with him the need for continuous language training and planning and organizing the steps that lead to the goals the patient has accepted. This process is found to be not only of great value to the patient but of equal value to the therapist. By working through the patient's goals with him, gaining a more direct and individualized insight into the self-concept of the patient, and planning the various stages of the therapeutic program, therapists find a greater satisfaction in their work. Rapport is more complete, understanding is increased, and success is more easily obtained. The patients soon realize the greater understanding of the therapist for their problems, their anxieties are reduced, and they come to therapy in a more receptive mood. All this reflects itself in the increased efficiency of the therapists and in the eventual rehabilitation of the patients.

Climate

The last paragraph touches upon one of the intangibles of all therapeutic situations, that of the climate in which successful results are most likely to be realized. The concept of climate has never been fully objectified. Actually there is a considerable difference of opinion concerning the semantics of the word itself. It seems of so much importance here only because the concept as used in relation to aphasia therapy is somewhat different from the one used in most other forms of psychotherapy. By climate is meant the atmosphere, the rapport, the bridge established between the patient and the therapist. It should be recognized that a good climate tends to reduce resistance, resolve anxieties and hostilities, and generally produce the maximal conditions for effective learning and personality growth. These factors are widely accepted as constant goals for therapeutic situations. Where aphasia therapy differs from other therapies is that, in order to obtain a satisfactory climate, much more than psychological ease and freedom must be obtained. While the psychological changes desired in the aphasic adult are in no sense to be decried and are of primary importance to the total rehabilitation of the patient, much more than the patient's internal ego needs must be considered. Many aphasic adults are in constant need of external physical care because of concomitant physiological and anatomical problems, for example, the very common hemiplegia of the right side, the visual abnormalities frequently seen in the brain-injured patient, and the convulsive seizures that so often follow brain disorder. So important are these problems to the well-being of the patient that for maximal climatic effect the problems arising out of these difficulties must be cared for concomitantly with the ego growth. In addition to the actual physical care, there must be real understanding of the problems caused by these additional handicaps. Thorough psychotherapy for the aphasic adult must in great part be aimed at reduction of the anxieties created by the presence of these real somatic complaints.

To establish the most successful climate, the therapist must not at any time overlook the very nature of the aphasic complaint, the difficulty in self-expression. This may be in many cases the major presenting symptom, and complete ease will be achieved in therapeusis only when a full recognition of this inability to relate to the human environment in a socially approved manner is recognized and understood by the therapist and that recognition is conveyed to the patient.

Good climate, then, as used here is that condition under which therapy is carried on which is established equally by therapist and patient and in which the needs of both are met in a mutually acceptable manner.

Self-Concept of the Aphasic Adult

No single factor has been so little discussed in the literature as the aphasic adult's own concept of self. Previous studies have examined extensively the neurologist's understanding of the cortical abnormalities following cerebral disease. An increasing number of articles and books[2] indicate the growing recognition of behavioral abnormalities commonly seen in the brain-injured adult as reported in Chapter 3. Psychologists have succeeded to some degree in isolating many of the thought-process differentials between the organic patient and the nonorganic. Nowhere, however, has there been a discussion of the patient's own concepts. Since therapy as proposed here is determined for the most part, if not entirely, on the basis of the patient's needs it seems important to establish to some degree what the aphasic adult considers to be his problem. Certainly it is evident that this plays an important part in therapy. Perhaps the very minor attention given to therapy for the aphasic adult in the past accounts for the failure to try to establish the patient's own concepts.

As the result of the author's close contact with diverse types of aphasic patients as reported in this study, it was possible to secure introspective observations made by a considerable number of patients as soon as they were able to communicate. In many instances these introspections were only partial; certainly, in the very early post-traumatic period, amnesia was commonplace. In other instances, however, consciousness was present almost from the point of trauma. It is believed that the understanding that came from the patients' discussion of their difficulties as they came to therapy considerably enhanced the recovery achieved. It seems of great importance that every therapist try to gain some insight into this area if he plans to produce a maximal climate, a thorough therapeutic situation.

The following paragraphs are extracts and condensations made from the introspective reports of over fifty aphasic patients. It is not held that these experiences as they are related are in any real sense generalized for all aphasic patients, yet a sufficient number of them were verified by their appearance in many reports that it is believed that they represent a fair extrapolation. From them, it is believed, a concept of the patient as he comes to therapy can be gained that cannot be obtained in any other way, whether by examination, test, or observation of behavior.

---

[2] Halstead, *op. cit.* Pierre Marie, "Etude Clinique sur les modalities des dissociations de la sensibilité dans les lesions encéphaliques," *Révue Neurologique,* XXIX (1922) 1–22. K. S. Lashley, "Factors Limiting Recovery After Central Nervous System Lesions," *Journal of Nervous and Mental Diseases,* LXXXVIII (December, 1938), 733–55. Z. A. Piotrowsky, "The Rorschach Method and Its Application in Organic Disturbances of the Central Nervous System," *Rorschach Reserve Exchange,* I (1936–37), 23–40. J. Eisenson, "Aphasics: Observations and Tentative Conclusions," *Journal of Speech Disorders,* XII (September, 1947), 291–92. Ward C. Halstead, "Behavioral Effects of Lesions of the Frontal Lobes in Man," *Archives of Neurology and Psychiatry,* XXXII (October, 1939), 780–83. K. Goldstein, *Aftereffects of Brain Injuries in War* (New York: Grune & Stratton, Inc., 1942).

Many patients recalled that immediately after cerebral injury or accident they had little or no contact with the world around them. They were unconcerned with the world and even with their ailments; they were awake only to eat and to carry on life's functions. Many reported that even these acts were performed in the early stages in a semiconscious state. About the only stimulus they responded to was that of light; even pain was absent. The doctor's needle during medication, or the feeding tube, if it was used, was neither pleasant nor unpleasant. As they described their behavior, the only picture it conjured for them in retrospect, and for the writer, was one of a state of vegetation.

This stage can probably best be described as paralleling the stage of early infancy in the development of the child. No anxieties existed, no insecurities, no deficiencies, no world—merely sleep and an occasional somnambulistic awakening for food. During this stage their physiological needs were being met; their psychological needs were nonexistent other than in a purely physical sense; they were warm under bedclothes, they were fed, and like the infant they were protected and loved. As their physiological needs were met and excess supplies of energy became present, they went through an awakening process. They began to notice the world around them. Like the developing child or like any postoperative, postcoma patient, they appreciated the visits of the ward attendants, the nurses, the doctors, not because these visitors stimulated them, but largely because they offered some change from the comparatively blank existence the patients were leading. As this period of awakening grew, all sounds were pleasant. Speech for most of them was just another sound; for the greatest number, the speech of others did not stimulate them to attempt communication.

First attempts to communicate came most frequently on the level of need—need to attract attention, need to satisfy wants, desires. Usually these attempts were met with great approval, but most often they did not succeed in establishing a true communicative pathway, and soon they were aborted and discontinued as other more satisfying methods, such as facial grimaces and simple gestures, were found to be more effective. Experimentally, they attempted to move and found, many of them, that they could turn only one way. They felt no loss resulting from their hemiplegias, only pain when they tried to move onto their paralyzed sides. They found they could sleep comfortably only on the left side. No memory for previous abilities to move or to communicate existed. They slept more than they were awake, and they were constantly hungry and would eat voraciously.

One patient recalled vividly a consistent engorgement of food to the point of nausea, and vomiting after every meal. As they were questioned by nurses, social workers, and doctors, they found it difficult to follow a thread of thought or conversation. When pressured into responding, they automatically turned to gesture and facial grimaces. Again, they felt no sense of loss in their inability to speak. As they were moved from ward to X ray, to surgery, to physiotherapy, and into this new world they slowly became aware of other persons as persons. No questions occurred to them at first concerning self, their paralyses, or their language in relation to others. In many patients this condition existed for several months, for others only for a few days. As they became more aware of the environment and the demands it made upon them, they began to experiment with conscious attempts to make themselves understood. In most cases, it was extremely difficult to get over to others any but the simplest ideas. After a short time, only the most outgoing continued to try. Responding only when forced to respond, they became concerned almost wholly with themselves—not in any critical or evaluative way, but with very minute bits of behavior. They found minimal activity fatiguing, so they withdrew into sleep.

They reacted to slight variations in the routine of living. Delayed meals, tardy baths, and failure to turn out the ward lights made them momentarily irritable. The rest of the time nothing seemed to matter except the minutiae of daily living. They found it difficult to respond in any way to the requests of others. Most of the men reported that, other than for momentary and very fleeting occasions, they felt no dissatisfaction with their abilities, no real feeling of futility, no need to do better than they were doing. They became used to their daily routine activities, were not self-critical, and became disturbed only when it was impressed upon them that they must change. Those patients who spontaneously found some return of language did not feel that by extending themselves they could do better, or that it was worth-while trying to extend themselves. They used what language they had. Some indicated that they had more language than they used, finding gesture and facial change more satisfactory.

Many reported that the recognition of loss of use of the hand and leg gave them their first real comparative concern. They observed other persons walking, running, and generally in movement while they were unable to move in these ways. This led to some conscious anxiety. As they described it, however, this was not an anxiety about their futures or a comparison with their pasts, but an immediate day-by-day difficulty—a feeling of anxiety about their present ability.

Comparisons with the past and anxieties about the future came through other persons. Initially, for most patients, it began with family visits; then an attempt to visualize themselves in a world outside the very sheltering hospital became important. At first, this concept was too big to encompass and memories of former behavior led to no visual image of the future. The difficulties of life passed on to them by their wives, children, parents, and sweethearts seemed to give exactly as much concern as these individuals expressed. It needs to be repeated that almost unanimously the patients reported that their inability to communicate with others was of little concern to them. A few of the men did report a beginning sense of a need for communication and consistent, if futile, efforts to gain access to other persons through speech. It appeared that these latter patients were the most extroverted and the most outgoing of the patient group.

From these observations it becomes apparent that the factor discussed earlier of the therapist's need to develop goal-striving within the patient is of vast importance. Early motivation can be achieved, it is believed by the writer, only if the patient's concept of self is recognized by the therapist and planned for in the therapeutic program.

Most of the patients whose introspections are discussed in the preceding paragraphs came to therapy in a severely aphasic state. The therapist should not lose sight of the fact, however, that many aphasic patients come to therapy with only partial language loss. Therapy is frequently started in a single area despite widespread area involvement in these patients. The area selected may well not be the most seriously affected one, nor may it be the area in which the therapist would like to begin therapy. Actually, it is believed that the total problem will best be met when the expressed needs of the patient are met as soon as possible. If the patient exhibits needs that motivate him to begin in a particular area, it is conceived as being the proper approach to that patient to attempt to give him assistance in that area immediately, rather than to attempt to establish what the therapist believes to be the most important area for the beginning of training. From the patient's concern about self in particular areas of communication came the working principle that greater motivation, better rapport, a more successful climate, and increased learning will take place if the training program is constantly adjusted to the expressed needs of the patient—the area in which he expresses his greatest concern. Through following this principle, it is believed that the greatest gains are made in assisting the patient through restructuring his ego drives. Through his ego structuring and growth, the patient is assisted in his struggle toward a new equilibrium.

Spontaneous Recovery: The Concept of Early Training

A factor which must always be considered at the onset of training is the part that spontaneous recovery is playing in the changes being experienced by the patient. In an earlier section of the book, it has been shown that patients whose therapy started soon after the end of the sixth posttraumatic month attained a higher eventual recovery level than did those whose therapy began after the lapse of some time beyond the end of the so-called spontaneous recovery period. Butfield and Zangwill have shown that patients whose training begins as soon as possible after injury tend to show an even more rapid and complete recovery.[3] From these data it can be said with some confidence that therapy should be started as early as possible after the brain injury. This will mean that in some cases the entire recovery of function may well be due to spontaneous recovery in brains that have had only temporary disorders rather than permanent ones. It is felt that beginning therapy with these patients is not a serious error. In the first place the effect of the training process is, even for those patients who would recover completely although they had no training, one of overcoming any psychological gaps caused by a feeling of not belonging during the convalescence period. There is a real opportunity to offset the psychological trauma which may develop as a result of even the very temporary presence of an inability to communicate. Patients have frequently reported that they obtained a real support and a deep feeling of being wanted and of interest from the training process. All this enables the patient to regain a proper balance in his recovery.

In the same area, it should be noted that many patients recover communication abilities only sufficiently for them to meet the simple communication needs of a hospital or gross testing situation but possess real areas of difficulty either in some localized or focal language area or in their psychological development. For example, one patient seen some four years after his head injury, whose language problem had apparently resolved itself completely and who had made what to him was a satisfactory adjustment, was found to have an

---

[3] E. Butfield and O. Zangwill, "Re-education in Aphasia," *Journal of Neurology, Neurosurgery and Psychiatry*, IX, New Series, No. 2 (April, 1946), 75–79.

almost complete anomia. As a consequence of the typical lack of initiative of the brain-injured adult, he was satisfied with his language facility, yet because of his disability he had never become independent of his too-solicitous family. While able to walk and able to talk, read, write, and spell, the combination of his anomia and his family, as well as his possession of the many typical nonlanguage behavioral abnormalities, left him at the time of his routine examination, four years after his injury, a severely affected individual, seriously in need of therapy.

For these very obvious reasons then, every aphasic patient should be given a complete evaluative workup before his problem is dismissed. It should be observed whether a problem exists, even though it is not expressed by the patient, and therapy should be advised whenever any area seems affected, no matter whether it be strictly physical, nonlanguage, or language.

The advantages of beginning therapy as soon as possible after injury are manifold with the patient whose problem is likely to be permanent. With the success that can be obtained from the combined effects of spontaneous recovery and new learning, sufficient motivation can frequently be achieved to shorten considerably the therapeutic process for many patients. Even for those who show little or no real gain during this early period, there is a real satisfaction to the patient and a real meeting of his needs when he receives the attention and support of the therapist during this most trying period of his recovery. The obverse of this working principle is equally important to the therapist. The patient whose therapy begins at some considerable time after his trauma may represent the most difficult of problems even though his actual language loss may be comparatively mild. As these patients go through the early spontaneous recovery period and gain some small ability to communicate but never go beyond that level, they become easy prey for too-anxious and protective families. They are frequently infantilized or/and rejected. As their attempts to communicate fail, they become frustrated, exhibit more and more often, and for less and less cause, the commonly seen irritability, and even show the catastrophic reaction to simple frustrations. They become accepting of their conditions, and in many cases they withdraw from social intercourse and resist any overt attempts to assist them. As their behavior patterns become routinized and their disabilities are accepted by their families, they either live out their lives in some highly sheltered home environment or are shunted off to institutions where they can receive the domiciliary care they need. It is a major task to succeed in bringing these patients to therapy when it becomes available. Unfortunately this condition exists far too frequently. Even competent medical men have found this problem to be so complex that families are frequently advised to provide whatever care is necessary, but not to expect or strive for improvement. While this condition may have been satisfactory in the past, the lessons learned during the recent war indicate that many of these patients can be rehabilitated to the degree that they can again become self-supporting and able to live a comparatively normal life.

The two examples given are meant to be illustrations of the extremes, the patients that are dealt with properly at the earliest time after the injury to the cortex and those whose treatment has been by and large completely neglected. There are of course all stages in between these extremes. The best working principle seems to be that therapy should be started for every aphasic adult as soon as possible after injury. The value of the training program is not limited, however, or should not be limited, to its use with those patients who are fortunate enough to receive training soon after their difficulty; rather it is believed that every aphasic patient should receive the benefits of a complete training program. At the present writing far too little is known about the maximal results that can be achieved with the old aphasic patient—old, that is, in time after injury. Experience would indicate, however, that in many cases rehabilitation is possible.

Summary

The present chapter has shown the principles derived from experience and from the literature which were used as a basis for the rehabilitation program discussed earlier. In addition a series of concepts that are either new or newly applied to aphasia therapy have grown out of the writer's experiences with aphasic patients.

To recapitulate, the working principles that seem most useful to future aphasia re-education and rehabilitation programs are:

1. That the aphasic patient is an individual exhibiting both internal and external needs with definable problems both in psyche and soma and others that are truly psychosomatic.
2. That the aphasic adult is an individual exhibiting behavior which could only be the product of his biological inheritance, his early environmental conditioning (thus his basic personality), plus his brain injury and its consequences.

3. That for the aphasic patient, unlike all other patients, the therapist must develop a special attitude toward goals, goal-seeking drives, and goal attainment.

4. That in aphasia therapy there must be a more broadly conceived attitude toward and development of therapeutic climate because of the very widespread nature of the aphasic patient's generalized problems.

5. That in aphasia therapy there must be a recognition of the fact that therapy should begin as soon as possible after the causative trauma. A corollary of this concept is, however, that aphasia therapy should be attempted for every case, regardless of the amount of time that has elapsed since the traumatic onset.

6. That it is necessary for the therapist to gain a thorough knowledge of the self-concept of the patient. It was pointed out that previously therapy had always been started with and aimed at the concept of the therapist concerning the patient rather than the patient's concept of himself. This earlier viewpoint is held to be an invalid one, since the patient's attitude toward himself is shown to be different from the therapist's conception of his difficulty.

From this theoretical structure, it is apparent that many disciplines are needed in the recovery program. In the next chapter the basic needs of a good aphasia therapist will be discussed and some of the initial steps that he should take in beginning the training process will be described.

Chapter 8

THE PROFESSIONAL APHASIA THERAPIST

In previous chapters it has been shown that the aphasic patient needs a widely conceived therapeutic program. It has also been shown that resolution of the aphasic disturbance goes far beyond the previously held concept of recovery from a speech disorder; that a new concept needs to be gained of the changing personality percepts of the patients; and that learning (and therefore educational therapy) is involved. From this it would appear that successful therapy depends upon much more than the individual therapist; yet, in practice, it is recognized that most of the work that is to be done other than for the hospitalized patient must be by a single instructor or therapist. While this seems to impose a special training requirement upon the aphasia therapist, experience shows that individuals previously trained in any one of the three major disciplines of education, speech pathology, or psychotherapy can with little additional orientation and training become successful aphasia therapists. In the following pages some of the general informational background that is essential from each of the three disciplines and some of the collated information from other disciplines will be presented.

Neurological Background Material

The therapist should be well acquainted with the common physical debilities seen after cerebral disorder. The following physical signs are seen frequently enough in aphasic patients to warrant their being considered as part of the general problem to be dealt with by the therapist.

Hemiplegia.—By definition a *hemiplegia* is a paralysis of the muscles of the upper and lower extremities on one side of the body resulting from disorder of the central nervous system.[1] It is to be noted that the condition improves with time but rarely is completely overcome. The residual or improved state is referred to as a *hemi-*

---

[1] W. A. Dorland (ed.), *Medical Dictionary* (Philadelphia: W. B. Saunders Co., 1945). All definitions of physical conditions were taken from this accepted medical dictionary.

paresis. In most instances where both the arm and leg are affected, the latter improves first and usually more completely. It is pointed out in neurological literature that this difference in improvement is due to the fact that the leg has representation in both hemispheres of the cortex, while the arm is represented only on the contralateral side.[2] Physiotherapy, muscular exercise, and occupational therapy are all advised for the condition. A realistic program, however, plans for the training of the nonparalyzed side for fine muscular movement. Vocational guidance as well as psychotherapy should be directed toward an eventual rehabilitation in which only the nonparalyzed side is considered for total use. Left-handed writing is always advised early in therapy, following the technique proposed by Gardner.[3] Prostheses are recommended and should be obtained following orthopedic consultation. Prognosis for considerable recovery of the paralyzed leg is good, but for total recovery is only fair. Prognosis for recovery of the paralyzed arm is not so good.

Hemianopsia.—In many patients a visual field difficulty is to be found. Most frequently this takes the form of a right homonymous hemianopsia. This is a condition in which the outer or temporal quadrants of the right eye and the inner or nasal quadrants of the left eye are unable to function because of destruction in the left occipital lobe. The effect upon the patient's behavior is to limit his ability to see objects on the right side that are beyond the field of the right nasal quadrants. At first this disability may not be apparent to the examiner. It should be investigated, however, in every brain-injured aphasic patient, for the consequences of the disorder in the process of learning, as well as in the process of living, are many. The patient showing this problem may not be aware of the disability, may fail to receive visual stimuli placed too far to his right, and may obtain only a partial and erroneous image of other material that extends beyond his field of vision. In general preparation of the patient for his total rehabilitation, he should always be made aware of the problem. Vocational guidance should take it into express consideration, and psychotherapy should serve to offset the handicap with a realistic viewpoint toward it. The condition is irreversible. Naturally, prognosis for the condition is poor.

Convulsions.—The aphasic adult, like all other brain-injured patients, is subject to epileptiform seizures due to the changed con-

---

[2] Paul Bucy, "Organization of Central Nervous System Control of Muscular Activity," *Chicago Medical Bulletin*, April 30, 1949, p. 838.
[3] Warren Gardner, *Left-handed Writing* (Danville, Ill.: Interstate Press, 1945).

dition in his cortex. The forms the seizures take are largely the same as in other patients suffering from so-called "epilepsy." One sees the *petit mal* attacks in which there is a momentary loss of contact only. In these periods even the patient may be unaware of the process. Disconnection in thought and in speech, however, may be the result. Too often the condition is overlooked, and the patient is said to be inattentive or lacking in the ability to concentrate or pay attention to the stimuli being presented. The more easily recognized *grand mal* attacks are also frequently seen. As in other patients, this type of attack takes the form of a complete loss of consciousness. There may be a preattack "aura" in which the patient recognizes that he is about to black out. In the attack itself, especially in the paralyzed patient, it may be noted that the first symptom is a twitching in the paralyzed member, usually in the foot. This reaction is seen to progress upward. The paralyzed side twitches and turns, the upper extremity is affected, and finally there is a complete loss of consciousness. The patient usually falls to the floor, breathes loudly, and becomes spastic, especially on the paralyzed side. He may bite his tongue, grip his hands spastically, and turn somewhat blue in color. When this unilateral activity characterizes the disorder, it is commonly called *Jacksonian epilepsy,* after Hughlings Jackson, the great English neurologist, who first described it.

Anyone likely to be present during a convulsion should be aware of the condition. If it is possible before the patient falls to the floor, he should be supported and eased into a comfortable position where he is least likely to hurt himself. If he falls before this can be done, his limbs should be straightened, something large and not shatterable should be placed between the teeth to avoid biting the tongue or lips, and something soft, if possible, placed between the hands so that the patient will not produce lacerations by the spastic grip. The patient's collar and other clothes which are tight and appear to be binding him should be loosened. Attempts should not be made to hold him down or to relieve his spastic condition; this must occur naturally. Otherwise the patient should be left alone. Since he has lost consciousness, nothing said to him is of avail. If a medical consultant is available, he should be notified immediately. Following an attack of this nature, the patient should be made comfortable and permitted to rest. For several hours he should not be permitted to travel alone. Most frequently there is a postattack weakness for approximately a day.

It was found in the aphasic patients described in Part II of the present volume that the patients felt considerably better if they were given an opportunity to ventilate their feelings concerning their attacks immediately after their day of rest. By general discussion and interpretation of the cause of the epileptiform seizure, the type of condition that increases the likelihood of bringing it on, such as alcohol, builtup and repressed emotion, too violent exercise, etc., and the effect of medication of varying types, it was found that otherwise treatment-resistive patients would cooperate in the self-help necessary. In some patients it was noted that there seemed to be a freeing of language following a major attack. Treatment seemed to progress more rapidly, speech seemed somewhat freer. This was not general enough, however, to warrant the making of any conclusion or generalization.

In terms of care for the patient, it should be known that several new and useful drugs that assist in controlling the attacks have been discovered since the recent war. The electroencephalograph in the hands of a trained and competent technician has been found to be unusually effective in predicting the likelihood of seizures and in many instances has been able to depict the focal area of any brain disturbance that might lie at the root of the disorder. Those patients whose attacks cannot be managed by medication may be able to find surcease through neurosurgical intervention. This approach has been found to be especially useful in those patients whose cerebral problems are due to direct trauma. Probably no single manifestation of the brain-injured patient has been and is being subjected to scientific survey as intensive as the posttraumatic seizure. In consequence, the therapist should be abreast of the information being supplied through medical research in many laboratories.

While direct treatment for the disorder should always be in the hands of a competent medical practitioner, usually a neurologist, the therapist must be prepared to explain and interpret the problem to both the patient and his family. A thorough grounding in the complexities of the disorder, the possible effects it may have, the need for constant and ceaseless vigilance on the part of the patient and his cooperation in treatment, the care and handling of the problem at home, vocational guidance, and planning and avocational advice and suggestion are all areas in which the therapist must be competent. It is important and should be noted that anyone suffering from uncontrolled epileptiform seizures should not drive an automobile. Vocationally it is thought best that work with machinery or in other areas where a seizure might endanger the patient or others should be discouraged. The prognosis for the disorder is constantly improving through research and medical treatment.

Facial Paralyses.—It is not uncommon for the patient to exhibit a paralysis that extends to the musculature of the face. As is true in the other hemiplegic conditions described, this is usually contralateral to the cerebral disorder. In the aphasic patient the paralysis is seen on the right side when it occurs. The facial paralyses seen were most frequently entirely overcome during the first posttraumatic year. Residuals of the condition, however, are seen for many years, and in some instances are known to be permanent. The effect upon speech lies in the area of enunciation and articulation. The speech disorder that is created is called *dysarthria*. The inability to perform muscular movements of the articulatory mechanism rapidly enough to produce the phonetic changes necessary for connected and rhythmical speech may be extremely embarrassing and frustrating to the patient. The speech problem should not be confused with cortical dysarthria, however. In the latter condition there is a tendency for the patient to reverse sounds or syllables, to elide difficult consonant combinations, and to stumble over awkward and consonant-laden words of multisyllabic length. In the dysarthrias due to facial paralysis, however, there is a tendency to elide almost all final consonants, to produce many words with the tongue held down giving the impression of consonantless speech or of speech as a series of disconnected vowels. This is important to the degree that the disability is affecting the patient's personality growth. It is commonly noted that the patient whose speech is markedly dysarthric and consequently increasingly difficult to understand tends to withdraw from society, or to become irritable and frustrated even more rapidly than does the generally aphasic patient. It is unfortunately true that direct therapy for the condition is of little more than supportive assistance to the patient. Psychotherapy and general balance in the personality may be of great assistance, however. It is fortunate that the condition most frequently resolves itself, for the most part at least.

It is important that the therapist be able to differentiate between cortical dysarthria and the peripheral facial paralysis type. It should be noted that emotional stimuli such as smile-producing humor provoke a natural bilateral facial response in the cortical paralyses, but a unilateral response in the peripheral disorders.

Medication, physiotherapy, and other physical treatment have been found to be useless for these problems. Time, encouragement, and psychotherapy are the only known benefactors.

Headaches.—Many aphasic patients complain of localized headaches. This is especially true in those patients who have sustained direct or indirect injury to the brain. Those patients who have had tantulum plate insertions and whose headaches refer to the site of the repair should be referred to a neurosurgeon. With present-day techniques it is frequently possible to eradicate the source of the irritation in a comparatively simple manner. Even when this cannot be done, it is often considered worth-while to reoperate to eradicate the source of the tension producing the headache. In general it is considered conservative treatment to ask for medical consultation whenever the headache is consistent, regardless of the supposed source of the symptom. Medication is widely used to control these posttraumatic headaches.

These five physical signs are merely the most common of many physical debilities seen in the aphasic adult. In the interest of economy it is suggested that the therapist familiarize himself with a more complete description of these disorders and the others covered in any complete neurological text. The emphasis given to these particular physical disabilities is intended to serve a dual purpose. First, the therapist must always remember that he is dealing with a problem that has its roots in a physical condition. He should constantly be aware of the physical concomitants and the part they play in the patient's concept of his own disorder. He must be prepared to discuss the importance of these signs with the patient and with his family; he must be alert to the possibility of an active neurological process which needs vigilance; he must be prepared to seek medical and surgical consultation and to cooperate in physical rehabilitation and treatment of the patient. Secondly, the description of these five common physical disabilities is meant to indicate some of the re-educational and psychotherapeutic areas that must be considered for total and complete rehabilitation. Likewise, the degree to which the patient is concerned with his physical problems as represented by these signs may well structure the type and amount of integrative training he can accept in language recovery. It should also be noted in this regard how much the physical condition of the patient establishes the mode and direction of re-education. A therapist not oriented to the physical problems of the aphasic patient is as unprepared as is the therapist unaware of the personality problems involved.

Psychological Considerations

Every aphasia therapist should be well grounded in the psychological concomitants of the brain-disordered patient. As an orientation Chapter 3 has shown the many nonlanguage characteristics commonly seen in aphasic adults. The list appended to the chapter is not intended as a check list of pathognomonic signs. It has the wider purpose of directing the reader's attention to the behavior implied, to the direction from which the therapist can expect abnormal reactions, and to the area in which psychotherapy can be most useful in the development of the patient's ego needs. No attempt is being made here to separate the areas of psychotherapy and education or training. Every psychotherapeutic situation must be considered as a learning situation, every educational meeting must be psychotherapeutic. In later chapters on associated therapies and therapists, direct application is made of some of the suggested techniques for handling personality abnormalities.

It is often necessary to work through a patient's behavior pattern with him. A recognition on his part of his problem and an opportunity to ventilate his feelings concerning it often assist him in resolving it. The repression of behavior which the patient begins to recognize as being unlike the behavior of his community and society may materially reduce the effectiveness of the recovery program. Evidence for this has come in part from recent research done with a small group of aphasic patients who were given sodium amytal treatments.[4] These patients were found to have a comparatively wide group of unresolved conflicts concerning their behavior and their acceptance by the people in their environment. By freeing these repressed reactions, it was found that the patients were able to relate more easily to the environment, that they had a greater speech and language facility than they were exhibiting, and that their speech and language potentials were less circumscribed than was indicated by test or clinical observation. While the research so far has covered in either type or degree only a small segment of the aphasic population, it has indicated that inferences concerning behavior patterns were generally useful ones. The aphasic adult appears to behave as he does in part because of a lack of knowledge concerning the abnormality of his own behavior. If the reported research is borne out through a wider application of the psychological techniques, the already recognized importance of thorough psychotherapy will be considerably enhanced. Kupper's comments on psychological concomitants after brain injuries in war are especially pertinent here. He pointed out that "although we may conjecture the organic deterioration to be vastly speeded by the injury, the instant mimicry of a serious state and its partial reversibility must be attributed to other

---

[4] L. Linn and M. H. Stein, "Sodium Amytal in Treatment of Aphasia," *Bulletin of the U. S. Army Medical Department,* V (June, 1946), 705–8.

mechanisms. We know that diverse factors which constitute character and personality play a part. . . . The almost automatic dependency and passivity needs of the individual become an integral part of the illness." [5]

It is suggested that the therapist be in possession of the accumulated knowledge concerning nonlanguage behavioral manifestations. He must understand the dynamics of the underlying motives leading to the behavior; plan to offset the abnormal behavior when it occurs; create a climate in which the patient feels free to ventilate his anxieties and tensions; be flexible in approach to all facets of the disorder, meeting the expressed needs of the patient as they are presented rather than working to some prepared and rigid outline of therapist-established goals. It is in relation to these observed behavioral manifestations that the therapist will find it most important to understand the self-concept of the patient as discussed in the previous chapter. It is held by the author that a patient's behavior must always be considered in the light of his disorder, his personality, and most importantly his own concept of his problem and of himself in relation to the world.

Because of the changing nature of the patient's behavior as he alters his self-percepts, either with or without the benefit of psychotherapy, the nonlanguage signs must in no way be considered as standard behavior, to be expected at all times. While perseveration and an inability to shift are commonly seen, there is a noted lack of perseverance. The patient reacts to the environment in many stereotyped ways, but as he changes and becomes rehabilitated these stereotypes become less observable. The therapist must recognize the patient's needs in terms of the changing aspects of his personality. Alertness to alterations in the patient's behavior patterns may well be recompensed by a considerably shortened recovery process. A failure to recognize the need for change as evidenced by the patient may result in a plateauing of behavior and the establishment of a final recovery level that is below the patient's potential.

To be eminently practical concerning the part that a recognition of these behavioral manifestations can play in the therapeutic program, let us consider these examples from recent experiences with aphasic patients. In the area of one patient's low tolerance to frustration, it was seen that structuring the daily lesson plan to lead to improvement of a gross nature in any area was resulting in continual failure and consistent affect-producing behavior. By the simple expedient

---

[5] H. I. Kupper, "Psychic Concomitants in Wartime Injuries," *Psychosomatic Medicine*, VII (January, 1945), 15–21.

of reducing the learning steps to acceptable and achievable although comparatively minuscule stages, the frustration was kept at a minimum and learning and growth proceeded at a regular pace. By recognition of the part that a low frustration level played in the behavior of the patient and the degree to which it prevented her recovery because of the self-directed affect it produced, it was possible to eliminate the cause of the frustration or to minimize it at least and to free the patient from many emotional blocks and consequently permit her to learn.

As another example, a particular patient's easy fatigability was soon recognized as a major etiological factor in his failure to show progress. The lesson plans, while not seemingly exhausting from an educator's viewpoint, were beyond the consistent effort of the patient. By reducing the amount of material presented in each therapeutic session to the point that it could be accomplished without leading to fatigue and consequent guilt feelings on the part of the patient, it was seen that learning proceeded in a regular fashion. By alertness to the changing nature of this particular physiological factor, the lesson plans were extended progressively until the patient was able to accomplish in a comparatively short time as much as had been previously expected of him in a much longer period.

The foregoing examples are intended to illustrate the manner in which the therapist's knowledge of the expected behavior of the patient can be of extreme value in the therapeutic program. It should be reiterated that a simple reading knowledge of the expected behavior is not thought to be anything but introductory to the therapist's understanding of the problems involved. Rather it should serve to direct the therapist's attention to the patient's behavior and to structure to some degree the kinds of behavior that he can observe and be prepared to meet.

Speech Considerations

Aphasia therapy has always been considered as the special field of endeavor of the speech pathologist. The reasons for this have already been stated. To recapitulate them briefly they are, first, that of all the groups interested in therapy of any kind, the speech pathologists have been most willing to undertake resolution of the problem; second, the initial diagnoses of the problem by neurologists of the late nineteenth century, which held that aphasia was merely synonymous with "speechlessness," structured therapeutic thinking and directed it into the area of speech recovery; third, the failure to recognize the personality changes and the possibility of recovery from the nonlanguage disabilities, as well as the changing nature of the behavior patterns, created a block toward directing therapy in the direction of psychotherapeutic goals; and fourth, the lack of recognition on the part of the referring medical investigator of the learning problem involved, as well as the arbitrary division set up between the so-called problems of education and the problems of recovery of language, created a condition in which the trained educator and the departments of remedial education were not even aware of the aphasic problem.

Recent advances in the study of personality, however, have stimulated interest in the organically disordered individual. Clinical psychologists have vastly extended their interest in the brain-injured. Experimental and physiological psychologists like Halstead,[6] Lashley,[7] and others have shown the beginnings of percepts defining the part that brain injury plays in the integrative functioning of the cortex and in the subsequent behavior of the individual. The concept of the aphasic adult stressed in the present volume is that of the total individual, where language disability and speech difficulty are present but are far from representing the total syndrome of affected behavior. It is recognized, however, that many aphasic patients are in direct need of speech therapy. Every therapist working with aphasic patients should have a working knowledge of speech and an understanding of the part that speech techniques can play in the total recovery program. It is recognized that this is an accepted fact by speech therapists everywhere, but the statement is included here for others who may be interested in the total recovery process in aphasia patients.

Direct speech therapy, as the term is used here, consists largely of the training techniques that have been found of value in re-educating the movements necessary for proper articulation, auditory training for self-recognition of sound constructs, and rhythm and voice patterns that are common to the environment in which the individual patient is to live.[8] It is in these areas that the specialized speech training of the speech pathologist can be of greatest value in the complete resolution of the aphasic adult's problem.

---

[6] Ward C. Halstead, *Brain and Intelligence* (Chicago: University of Chicago Press, 1947).

[7] K. S. Lashley, "Factors Limiting Recovery After Central Nervous System Lesions," *Journal of Nervous and Mental Diseases,* LXXXVIII (December, 1948), 733–55.

[8] O. Backus, in R. West, L. Kennedy, and A. Carr, *Rehabilitation of Speech* (New York: Harper & Bros., 1947). E. Froeschels, *Speech Therapy* (Boston: Expression Co., 1933). J. O. Anderson, "Aphasia from the Viewpoint of a Speech Pathologist," *Journal of Speech Disorders,* IX (September, 1934), 3–16.

While the foregoing may sound formidable to the therapist not trained in speech, it must be noted that many aphasic patients need little or no speech training. Usually the need is greatest in the very severe global or expressive-receptive types. For these patients it is often necessary to begin all training on the direct speech level. In most cases this is found to be a comparatively short training procedure. When it is extended, however, a considerable amount of time may have to be spent at the speech origin level. In the cases reported upon in the previous chapters of this volume, only five of the patients needed this type of approach. The second largest area of need for speech techniques lies in the area of the patient whose difficulty is centered in the sphere of translating auditory percepts into visual images, such as the written alphabet learned prior to writing, or into the spoken sound alphabet as in the prespeaking act. For the most part, an understanding of the role of phonetics is sufficient for this purpose.

The third major area of direct speech training in the aphasic patient is that of rhythm or rate of production. This is not unlike the area of eye-span in reading. The aphasic adult frequently regains communication skill in a word-by-word fashion, and drill for speed and increased rate may be found to be very useful. There is, however, nothing about this area that limits it to the field of speech, as though it could not be understood or used by other therapists. Many techniques have been evolved for the increasing of rate and the reduction of dysrythmia. These follow very practical lines in terms of the individual patient. Some have proved of extreme value; most, however, have had little more than supportive value to the patient.

Finally, speech skills have been developed that are found to be of value in reduction of the dysarthrias that so frequently are found to be counterparts of the aphasic adult's problems. These disorders are often seen in those patients manifesting as a part of their physical disability the facial paralyses that make articulation and intelligibility difficult. Unfortunately, therapy of any kind for the facial paralyses has been found to be largely futile. The disorder either is self-correcting and spontaneously overcome or it remains as a permanent residual. Speech exercises, however, may be found to be of some value in the recovery process. Many patients are able to get a feeling of helping themselves in speeding recovery from the facial disability. It is somewhat questionable whether the exercises themselves actually do make the recovery more rapid. There is, however, a decided value in the psychological improvement when direct training procedures such as these are used. The actual techniques developed for the reduction of dysdiadokokinesia [9] and the general dysarthrias due to cortical dysfunction will be discussed in the section under direct therapy.

By limiting to these four areas the discussion of the part that speech therapy plays in the total recovery program for the aphasic adult, the author does not mean in any way to indicate that the speech pathologist cannot or should not be more active in the total therapeutic program. Because of his training and therapeutic skill in the areas mentioned, it is felt that the speech pathologist may often be the therapist of choice. With the growing tendency to stress the areas of clinical psychology, of neurology, of learning theory, and of basic biological sciences in his training, the thorough speech pathologist is probably the best equipped individual to step immediately into the role of aphasia therapist as outlined in this volume. The overattention that has been given to the aphasic adult's problem in the past as a speech problem, however, has tended to make this the least important part of the argument put forth in these pages. There are many texts to be found in the Bibliography that stress the speech approach.[10] In addition, these techniques are reviewed at some length in a section on therapy below (see Chapters 12 and 13). The essential purpose of the present volume, however, is to indicate the over-all problem and to interest all therapists in the more generalized and wider problems of the aphasic adult.

Educational Considerations

Another of the major arguments of this volume has been to show the important role that the knowledge, methods, and skills of the trained educator can play in the recovery and training of the language-handicapped individual. It has already been commented upon that the language media found to be affected in brain-injured patients are roughly the same as the curricula used in many primary schools. The aphasic adult shows extensive disability in such prosaic areas as reading, writing, spelling, and arithmetic. In another context it has been indicated that the recovering aphasic adult goes through many of the same stages as the child in his earliest as well as in his later development. While on the surface there is a consid-

---

[9] Dysdiadokokinesia is the derangement of the function of arresting one motor impulse and substituting for it one that is diametrically opposite, or the inability to make repetitive muscular movements.

[10] See, for example, University of Michigan Speech Clinic Staff, *Aphasia in Adults* (Ann Arbor, Mich.: University of Michigan Press, 1947) and footnote 8 above.

erable degree of similarity between the child in the primary grades and the aphasic adult, it is important to stress the many and important areas of dissimilarity as well. The fact that skilled teachers can be of great use in the recovery process has not only been previously indicated, but research data have also been offered that show the effectiveness of their use in the program discussed in Part II. Remaining to be discussed are the type of material, the kinds of techniques, and the knowledge possessed by the teacher that are important in therapy.

The author does not intend to stress any particular theory of learning. Rather, it is suggested that the therapist understand the many theories. Hilgard's recent book [11] will show the reader the different ways in which the learning process is conceived by leading educators and educational psychologists. In this book Hilgard differentiates two major groupings of the field of learning theory: the associationists, including Thorndike, Hull, Skinner, and others, and the field theorists following Koffka, Lewin, and so forth. If a particular theory is necessary before learning can be understood in the aphasic patient, suffice it to say that the present author leans toward the latter group and the Gestalt theories of learning. The behavior of aphasic patients as they recover from their disabilities seems to be in stages that most closely represent the obtaining of a series of Gestalts. The accumulation of knowledge, the repetition of word drills, and vocabulary building seem to play a very minor role in the learning process with aphasics. It appears that the aphasic patient learns by building up a Gestalt. As insight is obtained, as he is able to differentiate field from ground, it appears that he is once again able to recall much of his previous learning. His old memory is restored. His vocabulary returns, and he is able to communicate using his old patterns. Where these Gestalts and insights cannot be obtained, there appears to be a distinct loss of what Halstead has called the "central integrative function" [12] and a loss of what that author has defined as a "power factor" that blocks recovery, that in a sense blocks the avenue for recall or that indicates the loss of cortical tissue in that area in which the previous learning was stored.[13] So much for a brief statement of learning theory which the therapist must gain from a knowledge of educational psychology and an observation of the aphasic adult in the recovery process.

---

[11] E. R. Hilgard, *Theories of Learning* (New York: Appleton-Century-Crofts, Inc., 1948).

[12] *Op. cit.*, p. 43.

[13] *Ibid.*, p. 68 ff.

There is a considerable body of knowledge, developed over many years, concerning the most practical methods for teaching the different language media. In this area the therapist can learn how reading can be improved, the proper function of the nonparalyzed hand in learning to write, the many approaches to grammar and syntax that have been developed, and the teaching methods that have been used in number and calculation work. Since the skilled teacher of these subjects is already in possession of these techniques, it may be necessary for the therapist trained and oriented in either speech or psychology to turn to the educator for assistance at many points in the recovery process. Or since there is nothing sacrosanct about the arbitrary division between education as it is usually conceived and speech pathology, or between education and psychotherapy, the author believes that any well-trained educator can be an aphasia therapist through an extension of training and of conception of self. The actual techniques mentioned will in part be reviewed in the later section on direct therapy.

The Aphasia Therapist

The emphasis of this chapter has been upon the need for the professional aphasia therapist to be a combination of speech pathologist, educator, and clinical psychologist. It might better be argued that he need be no one of these three but rather be aware of and able to implement the functions of all three. Nothing new is proposed in this discussion for it is felt that, in any educational endeavor in which the learner must verbalize, the therapist must be in possession of the skills of these three disciplines to be maximally successful. Certainly the speech pathologist must be an educator and a psychologist; the educator must understand the function of speech and the needs of the personality; while the clinical psychologist, in order to produce the desired learning changes in the patient, must be equally well versed in language constructs (note the new importance that is being given to general semantics in all psychotherapy) and must understand the procedures leading to learning.

The Basis of Learning.—It might be well at this point of summary to understand what is currently felt to be the basis of learning. It does not differ because of the problem of the learner. It remains the same for the child enjoying his first learning and the adult relearning old skills and new adaptations. Learning, to paraphrase

Prescott,[14] must supply to the individual an opportunity for the satisfaction of (a) physiological needs, (b) social needs, and (c) ego and integrative needs. These three needs must be satisfied in the re-education of the brain-injured adult as much as in the education of the child. Prescott argues at some length for recognition on the part of all educators of the needs of the learner as contrasted with the "traditional" educational approach which aims to satisfy arbitrary standards established by the educator and not necessarily internalized by the learner.

To be more explicit, aphasia training must recognize the extreme importance of establishing certain conditions in the training process which will facilitate learning. This factor is stressed at this point because of the apparent danger that aphasia re-education will fall into the very pitfalls that characterize all so-called traditional educational efforts. In reviewing the methods used in the few centers devoted to training the head-injured after World War I (these were all located in Germany), it can only be inferred that there was a marked tendency to follow old-line, conservative educational methods. Teaching was directive, consisted in the main of repetitive exercise, aimed at the predetermined goals of the therapist, and can probably best be described as subject-matter-centered education.[15] No suggestion is given in this system of a consideration of the individual, his needs, or his unique personality. It is argued here that advances have been made in our knowledge of the manner in which individuals change and grow; that we must go beyond the skill of language; that the recovering aphasic adult, like the new-learning child, learns because his needs are being met, not because he is exposed to a body of knowledge.

Who Should the Aphasia Therapist Be?—To answer the question, "Who should the aphasia therapist be?" it is held that all three of the disciplines mentioned, psychology, education, and speech pathology, have very distinct contributions to make. In an ideal inpatient installation, the services of all three should be used. For an outpatient institution it is likewise possible to work toward a staff where all three disciplines can be coordinated into a working program. For the more widespread individual treatment situation, however, the staff approach is more cumbersome and less likely to be practical, even though the staff members are available. Only in

---

[14] D. E. Prescott, *Emotions and the Educative Process* (Washington: American Council on Education, 1938), p. 323.

[15] J. M. Wepman, "Organization of Aphasia Therapy," *Journal of Speech Disorders,* XII (December, 1947), 405–9.

times of war do we usually find concentrations of head-injured patients sufficient to warrant the development of rather grandiose re-educational programs such as the one described in another context.[16] At the present writing, several universities have continued these extensive programs during the postwar period. The University of Michigan, using the nucleus of the plan developed in the army hospital at Battle Creek, Michigan, has gone far toward developing an ideal over-all training program. The greater need, however, lies in the development of therapists equipped to train and to treat the great number of individual problems lying outside the scope of the Veterans Administration centers and the universities. Caring for these brain-injured patients most frequently becomes an individual therapist's task. To expect the patient who has suffered a stroke or had a brain tumor removed or through accident has had a brain injury to carry the burden of a separate speech pathologist, a language instructor, and a psychologist, in addition to a physiotherapist and an occupational therapist, is unrealistic. Until such time as centers are developed that will be available for the treatment of these patients in every area of this country, it falls to the individual therapist to carry the load.

Roles of the Speech Pathologist and the Educator.—In consequence it is felt that the disciplines now separately practiced should be consolidated. The author believes that a speech pathologist can acquire the skills and knowledge of techniques now taught as the methods of education. Since the author feels that every speech pathologist should be a skilled psychologist in background and training, certainly he can, by recognizing the use that can be made of psychotherapy, become an accomplished aphasia therapist simply by adaptation. The educator will find it not too difficult to learn the skills of the speech pathologist that are indicated in the re-education program. A more complicated training may be necessary for him to acquire the background of a skilled psychologist. Yet, for the future of all education it seems indicated that educators should lean more heavily in the future on the body of knowledge called psychology. There seems to this writer to be a general tendency in this direction at the present time. As the areas of psychotherapy and education draw closer together and the educator is trained to recognize the individual and his needs in all learning, it appears eminently practical to suggest that aphasia therapy can and should be a proper outlet and a proper interest of the field of special education. In this

---

[16] *Ibid.*

regard it might be worth noting that the study of recovery from aphasic disorders may very well be the site of considerable educational research for the examination of learning. Certainly, if it is true that learning goes on in the brain-injured adult as it does in the child, an exhaustive study of the manner of aphasic recovery might point the way to a greater understanding of some of the so far unapproachable problems of general education.

Role of the Clinical Psychologist.—Finally, the clinical psychologist, trained and competent in the behavior mechanism of the maladjusted and the normal in our population, can (it seems) with very little additional orientation and training become a competent aphasia therapist. The skills and techniques of both the educator and the speech pathologist are readily available to but rarely acquired by the psychologist. With the background of therapy, of learning theory, of practical experience in guiding and counseling that has become the major focus of so many of the modern generation of clinical psychologists, the techniques necessary for aphasia training are but a short step away. The possibility of opening a new field, where the need for therapists is so vast, the amount of good that can be done is so limitless, and the general returns are so great should not, it seems to the writer, be overlooked.

Experience During This Study.—To demonstrate the usefulness of these three (now separate) disciplines in the aphasia area, the author points to the success obtained in the study reported in earlier pages of the present volume. The best therapists were most often the educators and the psychologists whose previous experience in this area was nonexistent. With an intensive orientation to the problem of the brain-injured they brought to the program a freshness of technique and general approach that produced the results reported. Possibly by the very fact that they came to the program without existing prejudice or bias concerning the magic of speech or language drill, but with a tremendous drive to assist the patients in their recovery, did they succeed so well. From this experience the author believes that success lies not in specific skills or techniques, but rather in the therapists themselves. An understanding of the patient, the ability to establish and maintain rapport, the ability to motivate and to continue motivation—these are believed to be the prime necessities of a good aphasia therapist. His attributes should include the ability to overcome the lack of initiative of the aphasic adult; an alertness to behavior changes, frustration, and impulsivity; the ability to obtain and maintain a good learning climate and to recognize the self-concept of the patient; and the ability to structure the learning toward acceptable patient-recognized goals.

The author believes that the foregoing describes no individual with particular training or background. He holds that the same listing of personality characteristics should be possessed by the good speech pathologist, the good teacher, and the good clinical psychologist. From this viewpoint it can be seen why the author holds that the good aphasia therapist can be drawn from any one of many disciplines. The author goes even further in his own belief concerning the selection of aphasia therapists. He holds that anyone who can read and write, who can subjugate his own personal emotions concerning the handicapped, who can analyze his own learning behavior and experiences into their various phases, and who can recognize the eventual goals of each patient and the immediate goals that he must obtain as he progresses toward recovery can be a successful therapist. It is in this connection that the families of the aphasia patient and trained nurses can be utilized in many cases (see Chapters 10 and 11).

In summary it is held that there does exist a separate body of knowledge concerning the behavior of the brain-injured that should be possessed by every one interested in their recovery; that there are skills and techniques possessed by the speech pathologist, the educator, and the clinical psychologist separately that are of extreme value in a recovery program; and that all these skills and techniques should be possessed by anyone attempting the over-all treatment of the aphasic adult. It is held further that anyone who is a good therapist in the real meaning of the word, regardless of his particular training or background, can become an aphasia therapist with additional orientation and training, and that for supportive and additional therapy any intelligent interested adult can assist in the recovery program.

In the next chapter some of the useful initial steps that the aphasia therapist can take in planning an aphasia program will be presented.

Chapter 9

PREPARATION FOR PROFESSIONAL
APHASIA THERAPY

The aphasia therapist's first insights are usually gained through
the media of medical and personal history, family and patient interviews, and pretherapy examinations. In planning the initial stages
of training, all three sources should be used carefully and exhaus-
tively. In the following pages it will be shown how these resources
can be utilized to advantage.

Medical History

Localization Data.—The medical history should be scanned for
helpful facts. It is important to know the type of neuropathology
responsible for the presenting symptoms. From the data now available it appears that there is an improved prognosis in those cases
where the disorder was localized in particular parts of the brain.
For example, in patients seen shortly after the onset of the disorder,
the localization of the cerebral trauma in the right cortex indicates
the extreme likelihood that the disorder of language is temporary
and can be dealt with as a self-recovering illness. In no case in the
author's experience has there been a permanent language handicap
following localized cortical disturbance to the right cerebral hemisphere (see pages 28 and 29). Where the disorder has affected the
left cerebral hemisphere, it is important to know the extent of damage
in the hemisphere as determined by the physician. Localized cerebral
trauma in individual lobes frequently indicates the major focus of
the direct language disability. Thus, defects of the occipital lobe
most frequently leave residuals affecting the visual sphere; trauma
to the temporal lobe may show receptive aphasic signs; when the
parietal lobe is the focus of the disorder, the severe mixed type of
aphasia is frequently indicated; while frontal lobe disorders often
affect the expressive signs in language and cause the loss of power
in abstraction and in other factors brought out by Halstead in his
careful survey of brain-injured patients.[1] It should be noted in this

---
[1] Ward C. Halstead, *Brain and Intelligence* (Chicago: University of Chicago
Press, 1947).

connection, however, that no such limiting localized viewpoint of aphasic disorders is possible for the careful therapist. In the author's experience these suggested signs are at best *only slightly suggestive* and not in any sense to be used as diagnostic of the type of disorders that will be found by thorough evaluation. At most they should be used as suggestions or directions that will be useful in first consideration of the patients. The electroencephalogram may be of assistance in localizing the brain trauma; it is also often extremely helpful in prognosticating the likelihood of clinical seizures.

Postoperative Condition and Behavior.—The medical record will also be found useful in its indication of the presence of concomitant paralyses of the extremities, of facial paralyses, and of other physical disabilities, the presence of existing needs for medication, the physician's recommendations for physiotherapy, and the early postoperative condition and behavior of the patient. All these factors need to be considered in planning the therapeutic program. The paralyses will indicate the need for training the patient in use of the nonparalyzed upper extremity for fine muscular activity. The loss of ability to use the lower extremity may indicate the need for exercise in the early stages of training and later insistence on walking. The presence of facial paralysis may indicate the presence of peripheral dysarthria or articulatory difficulty that will have to be counteracted in therapy. Medication and its importance in many instances need to be explained to the family and to the patient. Finally, the immediate postoperative behavior of the patient may indicate many of the areas in which psychotherapy will be important. It is frequently noted that the behavior patterns which become characteristic of the patient are formed in the hospital soon after the immediate return to consciousness. As a case in point, one patient whose previous personality description indicated a considerable degree of tolerance for frustration and emotional events showed an immediate postoperative pattern of almost lightning-like frustration to exertion stimuli of any kind. Recognizing this factor, it was seen that later direct interviews and examinations needed to be planned to minimize the effects of this frustration pattern even before the patient was seen therapeutically for the first time (see Chapter 10).

While a considerable amount of the material gained from the medical history can be obtained from other sources or will appear in later examinations and in therapy, it is wise to be forewarned and consequently prepared to discuss the patient's problem with him and with his family as soon as possible. It must be remembered, however, that the medical history is a very limited source of material for a final judgment on the prognosis of any aphasic disturbance. As yet insufficient evidence is at hand to indicate any high correlation between these data and the final recovery potential of the aphasic patient.

Pretraumatic History

The therapist will find many points of extreme importance in the patient's premorbid history and should secure whenever possible a thorough social service history of the patient's background. This material should cover such areas as (a) educational background, (b) vocational pattern, (c) avocational interests, (d) family relationships, and (e) psychological and other test material available. Each of these areas can be of great importance in understanding the man that the patient was prior to his cerebral disability. It has been shown in an earlier section that there is a close relationship between the prognosis of the individual patient and the premorbid intellectual state, while in another context the concept has been developed that the posttraumatic personality is thought to be an extension of the basic personality.

To show the value of the extensive history advised in the preceding paragraph, let us consider each of the areas separately.

Educational History.—Planning therapy for the high school graduate or college graduate is different in many respects from planning for the individual whose previous educational experience was more limited. For example, a patient whose history indicated a wide academic background was found to be stimulated only by material which approached his pretraumatic interests and educational pattern. Elementary language re-education that began with sight recognition of simple vocabulary forms had to be discarded in order to maintain motivation for continuous effort. Upon a recognition of this factor and a consequent shift to material on a more complex language level, interest was maintained easily and learning proceeded more rapidly. Further, it has been shown in the data reported earlier that there is a positive correlation between the pretraumatic educational level and the eventual recovery level in the specific language areas. The goals in re-education can be established best only by a thorough knowledge of these factors in the background.

Still one other point remains in this area. It is the argument of the present writer that aphasia re-education is not a matter of teaching a new vocabulary, new reading, new spelling, etc., but rather a reopening of the pathways leading to the previous learning of the individual. What is expected is recall of previously learned material, physiologically repressed by trauma to the neurological system. With this concept as a working principle, it seems of utmost importance that the therapist should have a recognition as good as possible of the patient's former language ability in order to recognize a satisfactory achievement.

Vocational Pattern.—With a knowledge of the work interests and work record of the patient before him, the therapist can plan language therapy at a level of interest for the patient in areas that may serve to speed the recovery process. A simple example seems sufficient to indicate the importance of this. A particular patient whose vocational pattern was unknown to the therapist until a point well along in therapy was found to be lagging behind other less well-equipped patients. When the information was forthcoming that this patient had spent the greater part of his adult life working with horses on one of the ranches in Montana, it was found possible to stimulate his recovery by building a learning curriculum around horses. Reading material concerning horses was developed and used. Animals in general became the central theme of the educational program, and this previously listless patient became highly motivated to participate actively in the training process. This type of illustration could be multiplied many times. With careful pretherapy preparation the difficulties illustrated can be avoided.

From the work history as well, some important clues as to the personality of the individual can be gained that will prove of great importance in planning therapy. The consistent, steady workman, the provider, the executive, the man who shifts jobs yearly, and the intellectual, white-collar worker—each presents fairly characteristic behavior in our social system. The ways in which the patient met and faced his previous responsibilities are frequently signs which cannot be (or certainly should not be) ignored in planning his reeducation and his psychotherapeutic program.

Avocational Interests.—Little further need be said about the importance of this area that has not already been indicated in the preceding paragraphs. This is especially true in terms of maintaining rapport, of establishing a working bridge between the therapist and patient, as well as in finding a core of interesting material upon which to base the daily lesson material. In passing it should be said that nothing pleases the man interested in active sports more than to discuss those sports, and nothing displeases the man interested in nonactive recreation more than a discussion of them. To the avid baseball fan, baseball is a never-ending source of material; to the chess player, baseball is frequently anathema. Any information on the patient's previous hobbies should be found useful in increasing motivation.

Family Relationships.—The patient's position in the family constellation and his relations to the members of his family are frequently the most important part of his history. The youngest child of a large family ordinarily receives in intrafamily behavior treatment different from that accorded the only child. The dependent younger son needs an educational and psychological approach different from that for the wage-earning father of a family. The patient's marital status is also of great importance. In younger patients it was noted that the presence in the family of small and dependent children often produced an area of anxiety for the patient that needed a direct and workable solution. The presence of a dissatisfied and anxious wife served to create an almost unmanageable therapeutic situation for one patient until his wife was brought into the situation. With guidance and some training she became one of the greatest factors in the patient's recovery. In other instances it was found that the high degree of emotion precipitated by the patient's handicapped appearance made the family completely unreliable and therapy needed to be planned that eliminated their cooperation. While most families desire to be helpful and frequently try to assist in every way possible, it is often found to be impractical because of either their oversolicitousness, their deep and unmistakable concern over the patient, or their subconscious rejection of him in his handicapped state. A careful investigation of the family and the patient's relationships in it is often repaid many times in the therapeutic process.

Psychological and Other Test Materials Available.—Whenever possible, the therapist will find it advantageous to obtain a picture as clear as possible of the pretraumatic intellectual characteristics and personality profile of his patients. In regard to the first of these, the data reported in Chapter 6 will be found useful. The expectancy in a patient of previously high intellectual potential is actually no greater, but the level upon which he can best be taught is decidedly different from the level of teaching available for the individual of lower intellectual attainment. A sufficiently significant positive relationship was found between the pretraumatic intelligence test scores and the posttraumatic test scores to indicate that some prognostic value lies in making that type of comparison as soon as possible.

There remains the value to be obtained from the measurements or observations made on the patient's pretraumatic personality. This has been discussed at some length in an earlier section. To recapitulate briefly, it is felt that the basic personality features of an individual do not change as the result of head injury, but rather that his method of expressing his needs and drives may change. He may be more impulsive in his behavior or more withdrawn, but most frequently he will follow the pattern set down in his earlier life through his biological inheritance and his environmental conditioning. All his behavior must be judged in terms of his basic personality. It cannot be repeated too often, in the writer's opinion, that a characteristic brain-injured personality does not exist; rather there are many personality characteristics that are observable in patients who have suffered from cerebral disorders, while the basic drives persist in a magnified form.

The Initial Interviews

The therapist's first contacts with a patient are often most important to the success of therapy. Not only is the therapist able to gain some impression of the severity of the disorder which the patient exhibits, but the patient forms many persistent impressions of the therapist. It is advisable that the initial contact should not be one of examination. Since aphasia therapy is frequently a long-term process, it is essential that it begin with a meeting of minds rather than a contest, which any form of examination most often becomes. In the patient whose language defect is only partial, it is possible to establish from the very beginning an understanding of the goals the therapist carries into the therapeutic situation. It is also possible to gain some idea of the patient's self-concept. The importance of this has already been indicated in a previous chapter. It is considered important enough by the writer that it is stressed here again.

The patient's report of his own condition, his attitudes and feelings toward therapy, the world he lives in, and his drive toward recovery may set the stage for the climate that is so important in the training program. These interviews, if properly conducted, can be as revealing as any amount of written history or opinion by others. It has already been stated that the writer believes that successful therapy with aphasic adults is largely dependent upon the therapist's ability to relate himself to the patient, by a free and accepting attitude, a display of warm understanding of the patient's viewpoint of self, and an understanding of the important part that the nonlanguage behavior of the patient plays in the recovery process. These characteristics of the therapist are on display for the first time in the initial interviews, they cannot be simulated, the patient recognizes their presence or their absence, and the course of therapy takes the tone of this first interview.

Self-Expression by the Patient.—The aphasia therapist must know that the patient needs an opportunity to express himself and must be permitted to do so in any way that he finds useful. He must often not only be permitted to give vent to his feelings and attitudes but often must be encouraged and urged to do so. It is often found advisable in an early interview to explain to the patient the meaning of therapy and the goals that are expected. In this regard the therapist must always remember that the patient is frequently unaware of his true physical condition and often of the cause of his disorder. The patient must be accepted as he is. He should know, if he desires it, the possibilities inherent in an educational program. He should be stimulated to make the effort *on his level* to express himself freely. The therapist must be as understanding as possible of every effort he makes to communicate. He must not frustrate him, but also he must not be too helpful. In this latter regard, it should be remembered that aphasic adults, like most people, like to express themselves; assistance should be given only when the patient evidences a desire for assistance or appears to be withdrawing because of a failure to express himself meaningfully.

Judging the Patient's Attitudes and Capacity.—The alert clinician needs to be able to define in his own mind the degree of receptive defect present, or in other words the degree to which the patient is able to understand what is said to him. He should be able to judge the amount of deterioration present and the consequent inability to follow verbal communication attempts. Explanations that are verbose, sentences that are long and that need considerable attention and concentration on the patient's part are most often frustrating and disturbing to the patient. Many patients have reported the extreme difficulty that they had in listening to lengthy perorations about their condition by well-meaning physicians, psychologists, nurses, and other hospital personnel. For the most part these attempts at communication left them confused, depressed, and unable to accept therapy. It is wise to keep the initial interviews short, to let the patient do most of the communicating, and whenever possible, and sometimes even when it seems impossible, to agree with and to accept whatever the patient attempts to convey. The therapist should reflect the patient's attitudes and feelings only when he is reasonably sure that he understands them; otherwise he should simply agree with the patient. The therapist must be cheerful, but not euphoric; be understanding, but not sympathetic; be realistic, but not overoptimistic. If the therapist errs at all in this regard, however, he should err on the side of optimism, for unless he is hopeful the patient will often reject therapy. Realistically, at the stage of the initial interview, the therapist can afford to be optimistic, for certainly the extent of recovery of any patient at that time is unknown to the therapist. He should be reassuring and helpful, remembering that the only goal of the initial interview is the establishment of rapport, for which there are no rules and no valid generalizations; in consequence he should be natural. The good clinician, the good aphasia therapist, is the individual who can succeed in establishing this rapport without effort, without personal anxiety.

Interviewing the Patient's Family.—A second stage of initial interview should be held with the family of the patient. This is best held separate from the patient. It is important here to gain as much information as you can concerning the patient; to alleviate the most pressing anxieties that the family may have about the patient's condition; to gain an understanding of the patient's relationships with the family and their feelings and attitudes toward him. From these early family interviews the therapist can frequently gain an understanding of other members of the family that will be of great assistance in the therapeutic program. This is of course especially true for those patients being treated individually or to some degree in outpatient installations. It is often as important to establish good rapport with the family as with the patient, for the success or failure of therapy may well lie in their hands.

A word of caution to the therapist seems to be indicated: Do not be too knowledgeful, too optimistic, too cheerful about the success of therapy. The family must recognize the important role they must play in the program, the day-by-day responsibility that is theirs. Wherever possible the family must be used, but their use must be expeditious. They must gain an understanding of the expected non-language behavior and be prepared to meet it. They must understand the aphasic language disturbance and its correlates. The therapist must succeed in making the family into therapists if he is to obtain maximal results. In this sense, then, he must start immediately in his training of the family.

Examination

The third stage of preparation for therapy is the examination of the patient. For convenience this area is divided into three parts, (a) intelligence testing, (b) personality testing, and (c) language testing. Each type serves the particular purpose which the name implies, yet each testing area provides information in each other area. Thus, the alert therapist can gain helpful and desirable information concerning language function from certain intelligence tests and at the same time gain some useful insights concerning personality characteristics. The same broad knowledge concerning intelligence and language can be gained through many projective personality tests. In general, however, it should be stated that most tests of intelligence and personality have been standardized on individuals who were not brain-injured, and the product of the examinations must therefore be interpreted with extreme caution. Since language usage is the product of all attempts to communicate, it can be tested in a variety of ways; in a later section of this book, a formal approach to the measurement of language function will be discussed.

Intelligence Testing.—The purpose underlying all measurements of objective intelligence or the individual's intellectual capacity is the determination of his ability at a particular time to respond to problem situations. Since the very nature of the aphasic adult's problem limits the modality of his response patterns in varying degrees, depending upon the severity of his organic problem, the product of the examination may well be a measurement expressing the aphasia rather than a projection of intellectual function. With due recognition of this and other objections to standardized intelligence tests as expressed in Chapter 6, there still remains a useful area of intelligence testing available as yet to only a limited number of patients in a small geographical area, but promising for the future a much wider horizon for the therapist. Halstead's recently reported laboratory techniques standardized on brain-injured patients presage a time when these subjects may be measured with some degree of accuracy before therapy and valid conclusions may be drawn concerning the intellectual potential and prognosis for recovery.[2] For the present, however, there is little to be gained by the therapist from expending the considerable time and effort necessary for the administration of either the standard paper-and-pencil or the performance type of intelligence tests. For the test-minded therapist, however,

[2] Halstead, *op. cit.*

it is suggested that the performance scale of the Wechsler-Bellevue,[3] selected items of the Binet scale,[4] the Porteus mazes,[5] or Koh's block design test,[6] if administered with a proper disregard for the formal instructions and interpreted with extreme caution, may shed some worth-while light on the patient's functioning level.

It is thought best that, whatever the results may be, they should be considered as inferential only. Quantitatively they offer little or no valid information, and even qualitatively they must be understood and used only in the light of the language handicap. Probably the best use of the standard intelligence test is to gain some picture of the patient's pattern of response to frustration of varying degrees in what may be a nonspeaking situation. The author believes that this can be done in many ways other than through the fairly traumatic test situation and that formal tests are often poorly chosen instruments for establishing the rapport and climate that are necessary for successful therapy. For this latter reason it is suggested that, if tests are essential to the therapist's purpose, they should be administered by someone other than the one responsible for the direct therapy.

Investigating Failure of Recall.—One area of measurement has been found to be productive of many leads for therapy, however, that of memory or recall. It is known that all brain-injured patients suffer to some degree from recall difficulty. The usual pattern is the retention of old memories, especially highly personal ones, some retention of recent memories and less ability to recall events of the immediate past. In addition it is frequently observed that the aphasic adult, in common with other brain-injured subjects, suffers from either a retrograde amnesia for the period just preceding the initial onset of his disorder or in some cases an anterograde amnesia for events immediately following the occurrence which originally caused his symptoms.

Memory defects of any type may have a decidedly important role in the therapeutic program. It is suggested that during the pretherapy period or soon after the beginning of therapy, when rapport has been established, some estimate of this area should be gained. Most

[3] David Wechsler, *Measurement of Adult Intelligence* (Baltimore: The Williams & Wilkins Co., 1944).

[4] L. M. Terman and M. A. Merrill, *Measuring Intelligence* (Boston: Houghton Mifflin Co., 1937).

[5] S. D. Porteus, *The Maze Test and Mental Differences* (Vineland, N. J.: Smith Printing and Publishing House, 1933).

[6] David Rapaport, *Diagnostic Psychological Testing,* Vol. I (Chicago: Year Book Publishers, Inc., 1945).

often the first pattern mentioned when no particular periods are missing in the recall, is spontaneously reduced during the first post-traumatic months. When this is not true, there is very little that the therapist can do to assist in reducing the problem. This may be found to be one of the most difficult parts of the entire therapeusis if the generalized memory problem is retained. The specific areas of loss described by the named amnesic period also are sometimes resolved spontaneously, but this is far less frequently true. Again the author has found that therapy is of little use in the resolution of these problems. Some hope is held out for the eradication of these latter problems through narcosynthesis. Research on this problem is as yet unproductive of any satisfactory answer but indicates the possibility of some valuable leads for the future.

As to testing in this area, the author has found the Wechsler memory scale [7] to be some value, but far too rigid for general use. In consequence the Sall-Wepman organic screening survey,[8] developed during the war years, has been used. This test measures memory function in all the modalities. Its basic contribution is not original, but rather it is a combination of many items developed over the years by psychologists and neurologists for use in qualitative measurement of the brain-injured patient. While it yields no objective score, it produces a gross evaluation of memory in personal areas, old, recent, and immediate; visual memories, auditory memories, immediate retention of digits, form memories, and old stereotyped memories. In addition, for the patient who has some mode of communication, it is possible to gain some estimate of intellectual impairment. One of the major features of the technique is the administration time, which is usually less than one hour for most patients.

It should be said in closing this discussion of the intellectual potential measurement of the aphasic patient, that in the author's opinion the formal objective test of any particular area or of the general intellectual function, while productive of many clues, is not extremely useful in planning or carrying out therapy. Most patients are frustrated by the tests and offer strenuous objections to them. If testing is desired, it is suggested that it be delayed and attempted after therapy has been instituted rather than used as a precursor to the training program.

---

[7] D. Wechsler, "The Wechsler Memory Scale," *Journal of Psychology,* XIX (1945), 87–95.

[8] M. Sall and J. M. Wepman, "A Screening Survey of Organic Impairment," *Journal of Speech Disorders,* X (May, 1945), 283–86.

Personality Tests.—Pretherapy administration of projective personality tests is subject to many of the same criticisms as intelligence testing. By and large they were not standardized on aphasic populations, even if they do offer data on the general field of the brain-injured patient. The usual product of the tests commonly used today is simple determination of the organicity of the presenting problem. Since in most aphasic patients this is not a problem in itself, this product is of little practical use to the therapist. Such tests as the Rorschach *Psychodiagnostik*[9] have been used by the author at some length. The material obtained was so limited by the patient's inability to communicate that the protocols were found to be of little value. Again, the frustration of the patient by the abstract figures was felt to be dangerous to the establishment of good training relations. Since language and communication are the bases of the presenting problem, the Thematic Apperception Test[10] is found to be of almost no value, while the product of the Bender Gestalt test[11] is so difficult to interpret that little more than an estimate of psychomotor difficulty was obtained. Some research is now being carried out with the Szondi pictures[12] on aphasic patients. Initial reports of the use of the technique indicate that some valuable information may be obtained through this completely nonlanguage approach. A recent study on such tests as the Vigotsky categorizing test[13] and Halstead's use of his categorizing and form board tests[14] points the way to some possible avenues of investigation for the future. For the present the therapist is advised to gain his insights concerning the patient's personality from his observations made during the early stages of treatment and education rather than to rely on any objective measurement.

Language Testing.—Most necessary and most useful of all the areas of pretherapy investigation is evaluation of the patient's language ability. Objective tests for language function have proved to be most satisfactory. The therapist should be completely uninterested in any numerical statement of a general or specific over-all function called language. Rather he should devote his attention and

---

[9] Samuel Beck, *Rorschach's Test* (New York: Grune & Stratton, Inc., 1944).

[10] S. Tomkins, *Thematic Apperception Test* (New York: Grune & Stratton, Inc., 1947).

[11] Lauretta Bender, *A Visual Motor Gestalt Test* (American Orthopsychiatric Association Research Monograph No. 3 [New York, 1938]).

[12] Susan Deri, *Szondi Test* (New York: Grune & Stratton, Inc., 1949).

[13] C. Hanfmann and J. Kasanin, "A Method for the Study of Concept Formation," *Journal of Psychology*, III (1937), 521–40.

[14] Ward C. Halstead, "Preliminary Analysis of Grouping Behavior in Patients with Cerebral Injury," *Journal of Psychology*, XX (May, 1940), 6–14.

interest to a measurement that will show the areas of language that are retained, the amount of retention, or the severity of loss in each area, the major areas of concern about language exhibited by the patient, and the general classification of the aphasia presented by the patient. While objective statements of language ability are useful to have for later comparison, the more important factor is the intralanguage comparison for the individual. In other words, it makes little difference if the patient falls within a particular percentile of language function in comparison with a group of other patients, but a great deal of difference if he can be approached best through retained visual rather than auditory stimuli.

Likewise, there is little to be gained from a knowledge of the correlation between an individual's performance in a particular language area and his total ability if that comparison is used only for statistical purposes. In our present state of knowledge concerning aphasia and recovery from brain insult, no prognostic value has been found except in the area of general classification. That is, we now recognize that the aphasic patient whose language disability is largely in the reception of stimuli is less likely to achieve a high level of recovery in language than is the patient of the opposite general classification, the expressive aphasic adult. In consequence language testing has been found to be most useful for therapeusis when it permits an analysis of the areas of language affected, the major or predominant collection of symptoms on either the expressive or receptive side, and the general language or communication ability of the patient.

The Halstead-Wepman Aphasia Screening Test.—In response to these needs the author and Ward C. Halstead of the Psychological Laboratory at the University of Chicago have collaborated in producing a screening test for aphasia.[15] The test in its present form permits an analysis of the language disturbance, a classification into major type, and a good over-all picture of the patient's communication ability. The following section is devoted to the test itself and to the uses that can be made of it.

Using the classification system discussed in a previous section, the test is designed to produce responses that can be interpreted in terms of all of the various facets of language that might prove useful for therapy. By presenting stimuli in many forms the following separate language functions can be separately elicited:

---

[15] W. C. Halstead and J. M. Wepman, *Aphasia Screening Test* (Chicago: The Authors, 1949).

TABLE 20

LANGUAGE AREAS ISOLATED BY THE HALSTEAD-WEPMAN
APHASIA SCREENING TEST

I. AGNOSIAS
  a) Visual form
  b) Visual number
  c) Visual letter
  d) Visual word (alexia)
  e) Visual size
  f) Visual color
  g) Audio-visual-kinetic
  h) Auditory verbal
  i) Auditory music
  j) Auditory number
  k) Tactile
  l) Body (topagnosia)

II. APRAXIAS
  a) General (nonverbal)
  b) Verbal
  c) Writing (agraphia)
  d) Number
  e) Calculation
  f) Construction
  g) Ideo-kinetic

III. ANOMIA

IV. DYSARTHRIA

V. PARAPHASIA
  a) Paragrammatism
  b) Agrammatism

From the presence of a greater degree of symptomatology falling either under the receptive agnosias or under the expressive apraxias, a general classification into major type can be made. When there appears to be an equal amount of disturbance in both major areas, the mixed type is apparent; and when there appears to be little or no ability to respond, the patient is usually classified as globally aphasic in language. By analyzing the response patterns it is possible to plan therapy by either of two methods. The areas of greatest loss can be seen and attacked directly, or the areas of greatest retention can be utilized as a means of gaining entry into the integrative patterns of the patient. Sufficient frustration is present to permit some evaluation of the patient's response pattern to frustrating material, a very important consideration in planning a therapeutic program. The test is arranged, however, to introduce a minimum of continuous frustration so that only in rare instances is it necessary to use more than one period for the examination itself. The author has been able to complete the actual testing in every case in less than one hour. Since no objective score is derived from the test, its only function is to give the therapist a rapid overview of the problem rather than a measurable quantity score. Sufficient examples of all types of reception and expression are given to permit an excellent clinical evaluation of the general language or communication skill of the patient. The test also provides a face sheet containing all the important vital statistics about the patient and a diagnostic code and profile permitting the keeping of records that are useful at a glance. In the later sections on therapy it will be seen how the areas isolated by the test are approached.

The following is a case history from the files of the author showing how the test is used to determine the language function of a patient:

CASE—*Mrs. B. C.* Age 62. Right-handed. Referral diagnosis—aneurysm —postoperative; right hemiplegia; right facial paralysis. Examined six months postoperatively.

Agnosia:

Mild visual form defect (unable to perform on two items; on eight other simpler items performed satisfactorily)

Mild visual letter defect (delayed performance on two of four items)

Severe word defect (alexia) (unable to read items above second grade level, some delay at that level)

Auditory verbal defect, severe (unable to follow items without great delay, failing completely on two items and succeeding only partially on five others)

Body (topagnosia) defect (unable to recognize the simple parts of the body schema)

Apraxia:

General defect in usage (failed four of nine items)

Verbal defect, severe (failed to produce speech on twenty-one of twenty-seven items; succeeded on only the simplest level of speech production)

Writing (agraphia) moderate (failed on two of eight items; extreme motor defect due to paralysis of former dominant upper extremity; all tests tried with left hand)

Ideo-kinetic defect, severe (failed all four items)

Calculation defect, severe (failed all three items)

Construction defect, moderate (partial success only one item)

Anomia: Severe (failed on eleven of thirteen items)

Dysarthria: Severe (extreme difficulty on all four items)

Paraphasia: None observed

The profile of performance indicated a severe expressive-receptive aphasia with difficulty in many areas of communication. Therapy was planned to reduce the verbal apraxia and the writing difficulty first as the most seriously defective areas. Plans were made for introducing therapy for the other areas as soon as some freedom of expression could be gained.

Using such a language diagnostic technique, it is possible to stimulate the patient to perform in all the required areas at a single testing session. By close observation and a careful annotation of the outstanding modes of behavior, a fair estimation can be made of the patient's typical reaction patterns. For example, on the case reported, no fatigue was observed, there was little or no overt frustration behavior (that is, irritability), and catastrophic patterns were observed on only two occasions.

Summary

The therapist, having collected information concerning the patient from a study of the medical record, interviews, and examinations, should be prepared to develop a therapeutic program for the resolution of the aphasic problem. The medical record has revealed the physical problems that must be considered, the hemiplegias, facial paralyses, headaches, convulsive seizures, and possible need of medication. The interviews have given some insights into the language difficulties, the familial relationships, and the patient's self-concept and have posed many of the psychotherapeutic problems that will have to be faced. The psychological examinations have shown the extent and severity of the language or communication problem, may have led to some estimate of the intelligence and personality defect, and certainly have disclosed the areas of greatest immediate concern. With this information in hand, a careful review of all the possibilities is indicated. Further interviews may be of great value —with the family, with nurses active on the case, with the prescribing physician, with the physiotherapists, etc. Each case must be considered individually, on its own merits and within the limits established by the individual patient.

Chapter 10

ASSOCIATED THERAPIES AND THERAPISTS:
I. PRIMARY STAGE OF RECOVERY

Necessity of Cooperative Effort

One of the primary emphases of the present book is the need for cooperation between the different professional groups treating brain-injured patients. This is especially true in the inpatient setting, where the first and very important steps must be taken to insure a maximal recovery. Heretofore the role of the specialist in language training and in organic psychotherapy has been stressed. Yet anyone who has ever occupied that position recognizes the need for wholehearted and active participation on the part of the physician, the nurse, occupational therapists, physiotherapists, and others of the hospital staff. Equally important at a later date is the intelligent and active interest of the patient's family. It is a major thesis of the book that only a combined effort can hope to achieve the kind of results that are possible after brain injury. The total-push programs outlined in previous chapters and discussed in the recent literature [1] were all the product of the combined efforts of aphasia therapists working in unison with other specialists and with patients' families. In planning a therapeutic program, one of the greatest problems lies in securing the type of cooperative effort described as necessary for a balanced and complete training process. Most medical and nonmedical specialists and certainly the majority of families are intensely interested in what they may contribute. The author may have been exceedingly fortunate in always working with people who were eager to learn and to help, but it is believed that this condition exists generally and that if orientation to the problems of aphasia is offered, it will be gladly accepted. This chapter will discuss some of the principles that have been developed which can be applied by any interested person and will materially assist in the recovery process.

---

[1] J. M. Wepman, "Organization of Aphasia Therapy," *Journal of Speech Disorders,* XII (December, 1947), 405–9. Vivian Sheehan, "Rehabilitation of Aphasias in an Army Hospital," *Journal of Speech Disorders,* XI (June, 1946), 152–9. K. Goldstein, *Language and Language Disturbances* (New York: Grune & Stratton, Inc., 1948).

Two general situations in therapy are foreseen: first, the inpatient and outpatient setting where an aphasia therapist is available to coordinate and guide the process; second, and probably the more common situation, where no specialized language therapist is available and the hospital staff and the families must carry the burden without specialized coordination. In the interests of simplicity these remarks will be limited to the latter situation, although they apply equally to both.

The Nurse's Role

Convalescence from the effects of cortical disorder of any kind follows the usual course of recovery from a debilitating disorder. The patient is usually hospitalized and spends his early and most severely debilitated stage in a hospital under the carefully watching eye of his physician. The primary interest during this stage is his physical recovery. Here he comes under the care of the trained nurse and in some instances has the benefit of new nonmedical specialists such as the physiotherapist, the occupational therapist, the social service department, and the psychologist. These are comparatively new but expanding hospital services, found too rarely outside selected urban hospitals. Most patients' primary contacts are with the nurse alone, and it becomes her responsibility to assume the initial direction that is given to the recovery process. Again, for simplicity's sake, the principles developed for these initial stages of recovery will be expressed in terms of the nurse. They should be extended under her direction to all aspects of the inpatient period. While general suggestions will be made, it must be remembered that each patient is an individual and must be treated according to the needs of his own problem.

The Inpatient Setting

As has been said, the first consistent contacts that the brain-injured patient makes after his trauma are with the hospital nurse. It becomes her responsibility to set the tone of the recovery process. While other medical and nonmedical services may be available and may play an important part in the therapeusis, the patient spends most of his time directly with the nurse. In caring for the physical needs of the patient, she is directly responsible to the physician in charge; in terms of the patient's psychological development or language needs, however, she is usually almost completely on her own.

What she does, how she approaches the patient, her attitude, and her insights may be directly responsible for the type of recovery the patient is to enjoy. This cannot be stressed too much. The author has been fortunate in working with nurses both in the army and in civilian hospitals who recognized this responsibility. From these experiences he is convinced that the greatest number of nurses are eager for knowledge and that they not only welcome suggestion in specialized areas, but seek out special training when it is available.

Importance of Special Training for Nurses.—The unfortunate circumstance that this additional guidance and training have not always been available can be seen in the behavior of some brain-injured patients who, months and even years after their hospitalization for brain trauma, are still languishing in the initial stages of recovery. One such patient was examined after he had spent several months in hospital and additional months in a nursing home. He was reported to be severely aphasic, mentally retarded, unable to speak, read, write, or fend for himself. His behavior was described as being impulsive and wild at times. Irritability and extreme emotionality were considered as expected behavior. While partially ambulatory, he needed considerable assistance in performing even the simplest acts. His attitude was that of a markedly withdrawn and seclusive person who put forth little or no effort of any kind. On examination it was revealed that the patient had considerable speech, could read, and could write, even with his supposedly hemiplegic hand. When urged, he could dress himself and even shave himself. Unfortunately he had never been permitted to try. From the day of his trauma the nurse had succeeded in foreseeing his every need. Recognizing that he couldn't talk, she talked for him. Noting his difficulty in performance, she performed for him. Whenever he tried anything, he was forestalled by the actions of his nurse. As a result he withdrew into a shell, became invalidized in thought as well as in action, and needed constant assistance. The nurse, in her eagerness to be of help, related her evaluation of the problem to the family, and they, recognizing their own shortcomings, placed the patient in a home where domiciliary care only was offered. It was many months later, after considerable effort and family coaching, that the effects of the hospital's too considerate care was overcome.

This, it is feared, is not an unusual example. Our veterans' hospitals have many patients "left over" from World War I. Many of these patients are, even today, almost three decades later, capable of some degree of rehabilitation. It is believed that, had these patients been properly approached and guided during the early stages of their recovery, they would have enjoyed the same kind of useful life that many of the brain-injured veterans of the recent war are today enjoying. The hospital must set the tone of the eventual recovery, and the nurse must become the instrument of the hospital's behavior.

What the Nurse Can Do.—What, exactly, can the nurse do to put the patient on the highroad to rehabilitation? What are the principles that will at least insure the patient's maximal attempts? They fall into two different categories, the first of which is recognition of the expected aberrations of behavior, the so-called nonlanguage behavior due to brain trauma. Following recognition, the nurse should proceed to develop modes of action that will offset the behavior mechanisms that debilitate the patient. The second category is recognition of the language problem and the development of modes of action that will assist the patient in making the best possible first steps in overcoming this condition.

These are described as two separate categories as though they appeared separately in the patient. Actually the patient as a whole person is being discussed, and his language and nonlanguage behavior are inextricably related. In part he behaves as he does because of his inability to communicate, and conversely he has some of his difficulty in communication because of his new modes of behavior. The two categories are treated separately in this discussion only to make them appear more distinctly and not because the author looks upon them as being separate and distinct patterns. Likewise it should be noted that the discussion is structured to appear as though this behavior of the patient occurs only in the hospital during the early stages of recovery. Actually everything said here should be carefully read and understood by the family, for the same factors are equally important in the later stages of rehabilitation. It is true that they will be less important in the home if they are properly and adequately handled in the hospital, yet they will always be likely to appear and should be understood whenever they occur.

Nonlanguage Problems

Considering primarily the nonlanguage problems, it is suggested that the nurse (and any other hospital staff member involved) familiarize herself with the factors summarized in Chapter 3. While this is not a complete discussion of behavior noted in brain-injured patients, it does include the major signs of such behavior. Some of these characteristics are more important than others during the early stages of recovery. In the main, however, it is suggested that there is truth in the old saying "To be forewarned is to be forearmed." If the nurse understands the kinds of behavior that are to be expected, she can recognize them as they occur and ascribe the proper importance to them. While some direct suggestions for handling them will be given, it must be recognized that each patient is an individual and will have his own way of responding to the nurse's suggestion. Consequently, specific suggestions must always be tailored to meet the needs of the particular patient. If one method of handling doesn't succeed, another must be tried. In the main it will be the nurse's flexibility in her approach that will be of greatest assistance, not the application of some previously successful approach that has been tried with other patients.

Overcoming Lack of Initiative.—One of the most prominent of these behavioral manifestations and probably the most disconcerting to the novice is the *lack of initiative* displayed by a majority of brain-injured adults. This lack of trying to better oneself in the face of what appears to be such a devastating problem is too often interpreted as an inability to perform. It appears that the patient is willing to sit by and try almost nothing for himself. After some apparently half-hearted attempts it is often necessary to force the issue of effortful behavior. The nurse must be prepared to offer constant stimulation of many types during those waking periods when the patient merely lies abed or sits in his chair and seems content to vegetate.

The kinds of stimulation the nurse can offer are manifold. Direct language stimulation will be discussed in a later section. Other stimulations should consist of such activity as the hospital provides. If occupational therapy is available, it should be used as soon as the patient is able to participate physically, even before he is ambulatory. If planned therapy of this kind is not available, the nurse should be her own occupational therapist. Many fine books are now available that list activities for the shut-in.[2] Those items on which the patient can succeed with comparative ease should be selected at first. To be maximally helpful, the nurse should work right along with the patient. This will stimulate him to greater effort. While a good deal of rest is necessary, during the early stages of recovery especially,

---

[2] M. Ickis, *Pastimes for the Patient* (New York: A. S. Barnes & Co., Inc., 1945). L. Griswold, *Handicraft* (Colorado Springs, Colo.: Outwest Printing and Stationery Co., 1945). C. R. Trowbridge, *Feeling Better?* (New York: Dodd, Mead & Co., Inc., 1936). E. Stieri, *The Book of Indoor Living* (New York: Whittlesey House, 1946).

the nonresting times should be spent in activity. Listening to the radio or watching television is not considered a good stimulation. These are, by and large, spectator activities, and what is needed is active participation. If one generalized suggestion can be made concerning the needs of the brain-injured patient, it is his immediate and consistent need for stimulation. Without it a whole series of disabilities will appear; with it an equal series can be obviated. The patient who is stimulated to activity overcomes his lack of initiative and is less likely to show many of the other behavioral signs. For example, the stimulated patient does not withdraw or become seclusive and shut himself off from the world. Since this is one of the most difficult problems to overcome in the entire therapeutic process, it is important that the nurse do everything she can to offset it by stimulating patient activity.

Offsetting Impulsive Behavior.—One of the most consistent signs seen after brain injury is the abnormal way that many patients react to stimulating efforts. Prominent among these immediate reaction patterns is the tendency toward impulsive behavior. This unthought-out and emotional behavior can be so upsetting to the unoriented nurse that it warrants considerable discussion. The exact reason for unthinking, impulsive behavior is not well known, but that it occurs frequently after brain injury has been noted by almost every investigator.

The behavior itself seems to be a failure to foresee the consequences of an act as well as an inability to exercise good and considered judgment. As an example, a patient lying in bed may reach for his glass of water in a perfectly natural way and then instead of drinking it may suddenly empty the glass on the table or on himself. One patient seemed to do a series of things that were designed to annoy the nurse. He would frequently throw the covers of his bed back and expose himself whenever a visitor would enter the room. Such behavior should not be a subject for exacting criticism or discipline. The nurse should make light of it. Chide the patient lightly and set about correcting the condition created by the apparent wilfulness. Such behavior is not malicious, nor done in an attempt to be annoying, but is due to an inability to control behavior on an intellectual plane. The effects of the behavior should be pointed out, the opportunity for repetition removed if possible, and the subject dropped. A continuation of the behavior will not usually occur if the nurse does not make an issue of it. Patients have been known, however, to act impulsively and later continue such behavior consciously when the results are gratifying. Too often such gratification is achieved only by the effect of the behavior upon the nurse or others. If the situation in the first instance is disregarded or treated very lightly, the gratification will be lacking and the behavior will not be reinforced by the reaction obtained and consequently will not be continued as planned activity. By recognizing the likelihood of such occurrences, the nurse can govern the opportunities for them to cause any harm. By assuming the proper attitude toward them their effect will be made minimal. Unless this is recognized, however, the nurse may find herself resenting the behavior of her patient and building up a mutual dislike between herself and the patient. These attitudes may serve to establish a distinct gap between herself and the patient and force either more disturbing behavior or withdrawal. The proper attitude will on the other hand entrench the rapport between the patient and the nurse and make guidance and therapy that much easier.

Dealing with Frustration.—An equally important sign of unusual behavior seen in the brain-injured patient is the immediate reaction to stimuli to which he cannot react satisfactorily. This results in frustration behavior, a turning away from the task or from other tasks, an emotional reaction, and at times even the reaction that has come to be called "catastrophic behavior."

A high frustration level is one of the most consistent signs seen after cortical damage. Some patients show it so immediately and so completely that only consistent control by the nurse can offset its damaging effect on recovery. In its simplest form it usually means that the patient recognizes consciously that he cannot succeed. For example, if he is asked to turn over in bed and makes some effort but does not succeed, he may cease all effort to turn over. Sometimes he may swear or express his frustration by exaggerated facial expressions. Fortunately, such frustration attitudes are usually momentary but they will continue if the patient is urged to perform the task upon which he has failed. They are usually not cumulative, that is, they do not build up from simple frustration to more aggravated behavior.

Being momentary reactions, they can be dealt with quite simply by the experienced nurse. As soon as the frustration is recognized, she should change the request or the stimulus. To illustrate, if the patient has tried to turn over but fails and acts in a frustrated manner, ask him to do something else that you believe he can do. As soon as he tries this new task, the frustration at being unable to perform the earlier task will disappear. Some patients dislike shifting to a new task, thereby leaving the previous act uncompleted. If that is the case, the patient should be assisted to complete the original task rather than to leave it. Completion of the task with the nurse's assistance will offset the frustration. What seems of most importance is that the nurse should not continue to strive for a successful completion of a task when the patient indicates his inability by becoming frustrated. The task should be changed as soon as possible, so that frustration is not forced.

The more aggravated form of frustration behavior is seen at times in a complete physiological and psychological outburst. This has been called "catastrophic behavior," since it appears to be the type of behavior evoked in a person when he faces an immediate catastrophe. It is usually out of all proportion to the seriousness of the task set or to the degree of failure. It has been seen in some patients as the result of failure to perform very simple and ordinary acts. One patient in an army hospital, when asked to name a particular object that was new to him, was seen to blush, sweat profusely, involuntarily micturate, swear, and throw a pencil which he had in his hand to the other side of the room as he tried to say the word and failed to do so. Certainly this was an inappropriate reaction to the task set or the failure, since he had been stimulated to name objects many times, had succeeded on some, and had showed simple frustration to others. There was no indication in this patient, or in other patients whose behavior has been noted to be similar, that the behavior was in any way related to a series of frustrations or to the severity of the task set for him. It seemed to appear spontaneously and disappeared almost as rapidly as it occurred.

The nurse should recognize such behavior, when it happens, as being common in brain-injured patients. It is not a reflection of attitude toward the nurse or other therapist. From discussions with patients who have experienced such behavior manifestations, it appears to be a completely unconscious act of the nature of the impulsive behavior noted earlier. Just as the nurse should disregard impulsive behavior and treat it very lightly, not letting it affect her behavior or attitude toward the patient, so should she handle catastrophic behavior. Treat it lightly, indicate its results, and go on to another task. The same stimulus should of course not be used, but another stimulus, one with which the patient has had a previous successful experience.

The severity of the problem is only aggravated by treating it seriously. One patient whose catastrophic behavior was not properly understood and who was disciplined each time it occurred developed a marked behavioral attitude toward all effort. It was noted some years after his brain injury that he approached life catastrophically. Each slight frustration caused a near catastrophic reaction, and many months of psychotherapy were necessary for him to gain a more reasonable attitude toward the events occurring around him. The nurse is in an excellent position to set the course of the patient's reaction pattern to new tasks that he may have to face. If she treats the frustrations and the catastrophic behavior adequately and correctly, they will not be psychologically traumatic to the patient and will drop out of behavior. If, on the other hand, the behavior is increased by continued frustration with the same stimulus, the patient's attitude toward problems may be established in the direction of frustration and his behavior patterns fixed.

Recognizing the Need for Rest.—The need for rest has been previously mentioned. Considerable sleep and general bodily rest are important and must be recognized just as much as the need for stimulation. It will be noted that frustration and other aberrant behavior are increased with fatigue, and these are probably the best indicators that rest is needed. This is especially true during the very early days after the initial trauma. But equally true is the fact that the patient will always rest if given the opportunity, and with continued rest there will be seen the already mentioned lack of initiative and tendency to withdraw and become seclusive in behavior.

The nurse has a fine line to draw as to the need for rest. Usually the need decreases with time, even in the hospital stage. By planning short stimulating periods in between planned rest periods during the first weeks and noting the tendency toward immediate frustration, the nurse can usually strike a satisfactory balance. Probably the most devastating advice ever given the brain-injured patient is "just rest for the next year and then go back to work." Alternate periods of rest and stimulation with planned goal-achieving activity constitute the only process whereby the brain-injured patient can hope to attain maximal recovery.

A good application of this principle was seen in the hospital room of a nine-year-old brain-injured patient. The room was a veritable playroom. Fastened to the top of the bed was a metal pole and suspended from it were a punching bag, a swing that could be lowered so that he could reach it, and a series of brightly colored balloons. As he came out of his planned rest periods he was told to raise himself with the swing. After he had gained a new position, the bag was moved in front of him and he was encouraged to punch it with his unparalyzed hand. The balloons could be pulled down, and he was permitted to pull them and even to try to break them. At the end of the bed was a fixed board, and a rubber ball was near at hand for him to throw against the board and try to catch as it bounced back. Everything necessary for immediate stimulation was always present, and every opportunity was used to keep him active as soon as he had awakened. It was an easy task for the aphasia therapist to go on from this behavior to stimulation for language. The stage had been set—he knew he was going to be stimulated, and he enjoyed the activity. Whatever is expected is accepted if it is made routine. Sufficient rest is indicated after brain injury, but ultimate recovery can only be achieved if the rest is followed by stimulation at the patient's level.

Insight into Concrete Reactions.—An important insight into the behavior patterns of the brain-injured patient concerns the recognized tendency to react concretely to present rather than abstract stimuli. This means that the patient usually thinks on a very concrete level. For example, a glass of water is something to drink— it is not wet, or liquid that comes from the river or a spring, it is not the material of the nearby lake or ocean, it is not the stuff of which rain is made—it is something to drink. The patient reacts to the glass of water as a direct stimulus that concerns him—not theoretically in any way. When he is thirsty, he drinks; the fact that the same liquid is needed to make crops grow, or that when frozen it produces ice or snow, is of no concern to him and doesn't enter into his consideration of the concept. He thinks concretely, not abstractly. Rainy weather, in terms of people getting wet from water, or a catastrophe in which people drown, is completely unrelated to the glass of water before him which he knows is useful to quench his thirst. This is an example of the whole level of thought of the brain-injured patient. Each thing he thinks of is directly related to its immediate effect and usually to its effect upon him. Abstractions of any kind are usually completely lost upon him.

This lack of ability to abstract should lead to a very definite course of behavior for the experienced and trained nurse who is attempting to help the patient. Every subject of conversation and every act requested of the patient must be put forward in terms of his concrete level of thought. It is futile to ask the patient to turn over in bed because the light for his attempted reading or occupational therapy work would be improved. The patient acting concretely would need to be shown that the light was better in the other position before he could grasp the relationship of his position to the light. It is useless to suggest that the patient would be more comfortable without a bedjacket because of the heat. That presupposes the patient's ability to understand a future relationship, but only the concrete suggestion of taking off the bedjacket would be meaningful; the results to be achieved by the behavior are abstractions until they are achieved.

This lack of ability to abstract extends into every act of the patient and must be recognized. Usually patients increase in their ability to abstract as they recover, and one of the good prognostic signs is the growth of the ability. It seems to be impossible, however, to hurry or train this process. It must follow from the generalized improvement of the patient's ability to integrate his behavior. Follow-up on brain-injured patients many years after their trauma shows that some degree of concreteness or of abstract-concrete imbalance may be a permanent part of their disorder. While some degree of concrete behavior is noticeable in almost every patient, it varies in degree from patient to patient and in many may be a very mild problem at its most severe stage. It must be recognized when it is present, and treatment of the patient must always be in terms of the degree of concreteness presented by the individual. In the very early recovery stages it can be assumed by the nurse that the patient will respond in a concrete manner, and she can then gauge the degree as time passes.

Anticipating Egocentricity.—Several other behavioral manifestations are common and play their part in shaping the reaction patterns of many patients. A marked degree of egocentricity is one of these. Most brain-injured adults show a tendency to be primarily concerned with events that directly affect them, but not even mildly interested in other happenings.

For example, one patient whose major pretraumatic interest had been in her family and in homemaking had as an early visitor her youngest daughter—age seven. The child was cutely dressed for the occasion in a new coat which was evidently her pride and her favorite possession. The nurse commented on the coat, and other visitors did likewise. The patient evidenced no interest nor any change of expression during the conversation. When the conversation shifted to the new bedjacket the patient was wearing, however, she became animated and joined in the conversation. Similarly, when the rainy weather was commented upon and the discomfort it occasioned to the visitors, the patient remained bland and distracted;

but when the temperature in the room and the patient's enjoyment of a warm, dry room were discussed, she again evidenced the greatest interest. Egocentricity extends into every act and event concerning the patient, and therapy must recognize the fact. Better motivation can be obtained at all times by referring every task set before the brain-injured patient to its immediate effect upon his condition. Discussing generalized material or planning activity that concerns others will usually find only momentary interest and frequently a cessation of participation.

Tendencies Allied with Egocentricity.—Egocentricity of the type described above is also correlated with a common tendency toward a lack of interest in the outside world, a withdrawal from previous interests, a narrowing of interests, and a general attitude of perception of the immediate environment as the entire world. During this phase (and it is almost always present during the hospital stage of recovery if present at all), current events in the world, the behavior of others outside of the hospital, the well-being of the family or of friends, the fashions of the day, or the condition of sick people in the hospital room next door are all subjects that evoke little or no interest.

Of equal unimportance during the early stages are future plans for the patient or the condition that existed for him prior to his injury. He lives in the present, the immediate present, his world is bounded by the four walls of the room, and his concern is localized to the simple task of resting and overcoming the obstacles placed directly in front of him. This narrowing of interest coupled with the egocentricity already mentioned may in many ways be a good and fortunate thing for the brain-injured patient.

Certainly one of the most consistent signs seen is the short attention span and the difficulty with concentration. However, if there were in the patient the typical interest in the world and the wide span of interest found in other people, probably nothing in the way of learning and training could be accomplished. Because of these psychological manifestations, all the attention and concentration possible can be centered on the immediate task placed before the patient and some consistency of behavior can be gained.

The nurse must take all these mannerisms into account in planning the patient's days: his interest in the immediate present and the immediate environment, his egocentricity, his narrowing of interests, and his short attention span and inability to concentrate over long periods of time. Basically, this means that whatever is presented to the patient must deal with something eminently concrete, something that concerns or is of interest directly to him, and something that does not require long attention or deep and lengthy concentration.

Evaluating Euphoria.—One other major factor of behavior needs immediate recognition. Most brain-injured patients are euphoric. This sense of well-being, of lack of concern or anxiety about self or about anything else, may seem quite out of keeping with the severity of the patient's problem. He will appear cheerful and largely unconcerned about a condition that the nurse and the doctor recognize as being devastating and debilitating.

This euphoria may be very disconcerting unless properly evaluated as a typical sign of brain injury. It is not an indication of a loss of intelligence or of an inability to encompass the severity of a problem, but is a very satisfactory and valuable condition. Without euphoria during the early stages of recovery, most patients would be depressed and anxious to the degree that nothing could be done for them. Anxiety and concern begin soon enough, and when it does the patients are frequently so upset and so depressed that only extremely competent handling can produce motivation sufficient to pierce their armor of withdrawal.

The nurse should take advantage of the euphoric condition. During the stay in the hospital, while the patient is most unconcerned and before the shadow of self-realization becomes a conditioning factor, the nurse can establish routines of training and therapy that become so entrenched and so much a part of the daily behavior of the patient that they are accepted and become permanent. This contribution, if properly established, can be the source of a continuing course of action for all therapy and can well be the determining factor in a complete recovery process.

Judgment of Intelligence.—Several other questions are prominent in considering the brain-injured adult patient. What of his intelligence? Does he actually have as much difficulty in remembering things as he appears to have? These are not easy questions to answer. Both intelligence and memory are so inextricably bound up in total behavior that it is impossible to give a simple answer. In many instances it will be noted that the apparent lack of intellectual behavior is more a matter of inability to understand the usual spoken language of the community; in terms of language problems, this is called a receptive aphasia. Or it may be apparent that the patient understands a good deal of what is said directly to him but seems incapable of making use of the information in any practical, responsive sense—and this is frequently the expressive aphasic behavior.

Often after brain injury intelligence seems to be spared, but behavior never again reaches the same level of activity that was possessed formerly. The concreteness of behavior makes it appear that the patient is less well able to use the common symbols of our complex and abstract society, which seems to be a form of intelligence. With the changed brain, which must form new integrations in ways that require considerable training before achievement can even be mentioned, there usually follows a different type of intelligence.

Probably the best attitude toward the brain-injured patient from the viewpoint of intelligence is that, in the early days of recovery at least, he is so preoccupied both consciously and subconsciously with the tremendous task of reintegration and physical recovery that his intellect is held in abeyance. He does not possess sufficient neural energy to use the intelligence he may possess. His learning and his recovery are dependent to a large degree upon the ability to form these new integrations. As he overcomes the physical disability, the paralysis which may be a concomitant, the neurological distortions which were formed by the cortical destruction, and the debility of physical weakness, much of his intellectual functioning may return. Intelligence as an entity probably denies simple definition. The nurse working with the severely brain-injured patient probably does best to disregard any consideration of the intellectual ability of her patient. She must work with him as though he were going to recover in every capacity. No one knows at this time which patients will be capable of a returning intellectual function at their previous level. Consider the patients as people who frequently need to start all over again, and give them every assistance by recalling all the behavioral manifestations as being part of their new recovering personality.

Recovery of Recall.—The answer to the problem of memory and its retention is a far simpler one when considered from the behavioral viewpoint. It is known and entirely expected that the brain-injured patient will have memory loss. During the very early stages after trauma, he may have almost no recall at all. This condition should get progressively better. Memory should recover during the early stages in somewhat the following pattern. Old personal memories will return first and will appear to be best retained. Do not confuse this return of old memories with a complete return of the ability to recall, for it may be the only memory area which will appear intact. Recent memories of things, events, and persons known in the recent past will suffer some loss of recall. This area of memory also may show progressive return during the hospital stay, but in many patients it may be a severely debilitated condition for many months after trauma, and in some it may not return at all.

Most seriously affected, however, will be the immediate memory area. Things just learned, the number of the room which was just repeated, the word that the patient could say a half-hour previously will often just seem to disappear from mind. Do not interpret this as a loss of intelligence or of interest. It is a common occurrence after brain injury for the immediate memory to be so affected that the patient will not recall where he is when he awakens each day. It seems to be of little use during these early days of convalescence to spend too much time attempting to get the patient to try to recall immediate events. That the things he learns are intact within his cortex has, however, been demonstrated. Many patients who were unable to recall newly learned material when asked to repeat it immediately were found capable of repeating this same information when asked for it a week or a month later. In this respect, repetition to show improvement is a futile task.

These seem to be the most important of the many behavioral manifestations that follow brain injury. That they cannot be completely separated from the language problem can easily be seen. On the following pages will be found some of the principles that the nurse and others concerned with the aphasic brain-injured patient while he is hospitalized can do to start him off on the correct pathway to rehabilitation. These need to be understood as specific illustrations of generalized conditions. They may not apply directly to any patient seen by any nurse, but by being flexible and shifting them to meet the particular needs of the individual patient they may be made of considerable value. At least they will show what the nurse may be able to do and some of the principles that she can follow in establishing the pathways toward language recovery.

Inpatient Language Therapy

Many brain-injured patients during the early stages of recovery from cerebral insult show language difficulties as a part of their behavioral patterns. Fortunately the greatest number of these patients show this type of handicap for a short and transitory period only. Most of the aphasic disturbances are overcome spontaneously during the very early stage of convalescence. Spontaneous recovery of this type is usually dramatic and rapid. During the very first days there may be a change from a completely nonspeaking, nonunderstanding state to a progressive recovery of all or most of the previous language skills. Even the severe dysarthrias, in which articulation and production of speech are so confused that it is almost totally unintelligible, may well clear up to the point of normal articulation within a week's time. The nurse need only observe the language behavior of her patients to recognize this rapidly changing condition. Naturally, as this type of recovery is observed, no therapy is necessary. The nurse will, however, do well not to press or urge the patient to difficult speech or language effort during this time, for frustration, withdrawal, and consequent psychological disturbances have been known to result from extended effort by even rapidly improving patients. Early recovery of this kind is thought to be due to the fact that the brain trauma did not directly affect areas of the brain concerned in language reception or production, but that these areas were temporarily affected as the result of edema or shock and that, as the natural healing proceeds, capability of function is spontaneously recovered.

A second group of patients will be seen who seem to recover their language facility to the degree that it was possessed pretraumatically. For all practical purposes it will appear that, like the first group, their defects were temporary. Close examination of all the language factors in these patients may however reveal a residual aphasia. That is, the patient may regain the ability to speak and read and write and superficially may appear to have suffered no ill effects from the brain disorder, but when he attempts to use numbers or to spell, or to recognize forms or music, he may find himself seriously disabled. These isolated disabilities may only be revealed by a thorough examination. The fact that they may appear in the presence of an apparently complete recovery indicates that wherever it is possible every brain-injured patient should have the benefit of a complete aphasia examination before he is discharged from the hospital. If a clinical psychologist or an aphasia therapist is available, it is suggested that a consultation be arranged prior to the hospital discharge to study the aphasic problem in all its complexities so that the patient and the family can be prepared for the task that lies before them. When such services are not available, it is still possible for the nurse, the doctor, or the intern to examine the different facets of language and make such a differential diagnosis. Language examinations such as those discussed in an earlier chapter are now available and are simple enough for any professionally trained person to administer, so that these separate language factors can be elicited and the family and patient properly oriented.

The third group of patients are those who show little or no immediate spontaneous recovery—if there is a return of language it is only partial—during the early hospital stage of convalescence. These patients require special handling, and the nurses and others of the professional hospital staff face a particularly complex task with them. Not only must they be careful to avoid behavior that will be deleterious to the immediate recovery of their patients, but they also have the greater responsibility of establishing for many patients the proper first contacts that will aid in the lengthy and difficult recuperation problem.

Certain principles of good language treatment can be understood and followed that will aid immeasurably the future treatment course of the aphasic adult, just as their avoidance or misapplication can produce long-standing problems that may delay and negate later recovery. As has been stated earlier, the observance of these principles should be the duty of all members of the inpatient staff, the doctor, the physiotherapist, the occupational therapist, the social worker, the psychologist, and the nurse. While each of these disciplines may face the problem in different ways and for varying amounts of time during the hospital stay, the nurses more than any other single group are usually in closest contact with the patient, and these remarks will be addressed directly to this group, with the understanding that they are equally important to the other groups.

Evaluating the Language Problem.—The first principle concerns evaluation of the language problem. To the best of her ability the nurse should attempt during the very early stages to estimate the type and degree of the patient's language problem. For practical purposes it is suggested that the first language area investigated should be the patient's ability to understand simple spoken speech. That is, how well can the patient understand what is said to him? This can be simply tested by asking the patient to perform expected tasks, such as turning over in bed at request or pointing to the window or the ever-present glass of water.

Automatic Responses. The nurse attempting to evaluate understanding of language should be careful to avoid accompanying the requests made by gestures or actions. These can be interpreted meaningfully by many patients who cannot understand spoken language. Also, it must be noted that understanding is not shown by simple verbal responses to common questions. For example, the how-are-you-this-morning type of question which is automatically answered by "Fine" or an affirmative nod of the head does not indicate understanding. Most aphasic patients have a small stock of automatic phrases or words or gestures which they use whenever they believe language is required of them or whenever they attempt speech. If they expect a certain question, they may answer it correctly with these automatic words and it will seem that they understand what is being said to them when they do not comprehend the actual context. Recognizing the existence of these automatisms, the nurse should gauge understanding by performance rather than verbal response, since of necessity the types of things that can be asked of the nonambulatory patient are limited and the automatic phrases are too often sufficient to answer these very simple questions. One patient whose automatic language consisted of the affirmative "yes" and the negative "no" was thought to understand almost everything said to her for several weeks by the chance correct use of these words while she was bedridden. As soon as she was ambulatory, however, and was asked to do something for herself, it was seen that she could not understand even the simplest questions that lead to performance.

EXPRESSIVE ABILITY. The understanding of meaningful language is more difficult to evaluate than use of language, the expressive half of the disorders seen in brain-injured patients. Here again, there must be some recognition of automatic phrases. It remains a much simpler task, however, to note that only certain words are used and that these words are just as often used incorrectly as they are correctly. If all questions asked, however, are framed to produce a particular response such as the brief affirmative statement, there may be some early difficulty in recognizing the expressive as well as the receptive features of the disability. Whenever the same word or phrase is used by the patient for almost any response, it should be noted as automatic verbalization and questions should be framed that cannot be answered correctly by using those phrases.

It is usually not a good practice merely to state questions negatively if the automatism seems to be the affirmative "yes." This may lead to awkward sentence structure and to complex sentences that are difficult to follow. To elicit language expression in its simplest form, show the patient who seems to understand language some common object like a glass of water or a pencil or a book and simply ask for its name. Naming of objects is the simplest form of propositional speech, but it does require a total integration of language, and if it can be performed properly and correctly propositional speech can be used and the cortex is intact enough to produce the integrations necessary for language.

Beyond this simple stage of expression are varying degrees of language complexity. Return of expressive speech usually follows the same pattern that speech and language learning follows in the child. Thus, nouns or common names for objects and things are the first learned patterns. Pronouns, especially the personal pronouns, form a part of the first stage but usually follow the actual learning and use of some noun forms. Verbs or action words are next and, with several notable exceptions, may be added to the nouns to form meaningful if ungrammatical sentences. The verbs "to be" and "to have" as auxiliaries are the most marked exceptions to this rule. Frequently these words used correctly are not included in the correct language usage patterns of the aphasic patient until rather late in therapy.[3] Following the use of nouns and verbs comes the use of modifiers, the adjectives first, then the adverbs. These forms are usually added some time after two-word sentences are reasonably well formed. The nurse, recognizing this four-part learning process, can gauge rather accurately the stage of development that the particular patient has reached.

The expressive patient, the one having difficulty in putting language into a spoken or written form, usually has marked difficulty in using the grammatical parts of speech. The very simplest-appearing words often give the greatest difficulty. In consequence, speech at first sounds, even when quite complete, like the phrasing commonly used in a telegram. Simple one-word or two-word sentences take the place of exposition of grammatical significance. The articles, prepositions, conjunctions, etc., may not be used until long after the patient has developed a fairly useful form of expression, and this is usually long after discharge from the hospital.

For practical purposes, again, the nurse should make as good determination of the patient's ability to use spoken language as she can. This will help her understand the patient's attempts to speak and will not leave her unprepared for the rather difficult process of understanding an apparently intelligent patient as he attempts to explain a complex attitude or feeling in one or two words. Most persons have a distinct tendency to attempt to assist the patient to try to use complete sentences when he is at this very simple language stage. This should be avoided, since it will do nothing but frustrate

---

[3] J. O. Anderson, "*Is* Is Not the Verb for Aphasia," *Journal of Speech Disorders*, XI (June, 1946), 175–78.

the patient and produce many of the nonlanguage signs mentioned earlier that are very debilitating.

One other factor should be understood at this early evaluation and treatment stage. The nurse should not be confused by the patient's apparent ability to use phrases and even some short and complete sentences at certain times and his inability to express his attitudes and feelings at other times. Some phrases and words seem to be retained by some patients, and these can be used accurately, while other words and phrases at what appears to be the same level of difficulty are not available to the patient.

The nurse should also recognize the existence of certain so-called emotional words and phrases. They may be the corollary of attitudes of frustration and catastrophic reaction. One patient, a woman of quiet demeanor and good background, always expressed her feelings of this kind by saying, "Damn it to hell" every time she tried something and could not succeed. These words apparently had little meaning to her and were only an unrepressed emotion being expressed. They did not mean that she could use four-word sentences or other words or phrases on the same level of difficulty but only that with her inability to cope with a situation she responded emotionally, and with her inability to repress these emotions she used words that were extremely unlike her expected command of language.

READING ABILITY. Having to some degree determined the spoken language abilities of the patient, the nurse should also attempt to determine how well the patient can read the written or printed language form. This is especially necessary for the patient who cannot understand the spoken word. Many patients have a limited aphasia that affects only one aspect of language and may retain some of the other avenues of understanding language.

The nurse should follow a procedure not unlike that discussed above for the spoken word—showing the patient a single naming word printed in large letters on a plain sheet of paper and trying to elicit a spoken response. As the word is shown, she should ask the patient what it says. If oral language is difficult because of an expressive aphasia, the word is shown and then the patient is asked to point to the named article in the room. If this type of communication can be established, it will open some avenues for later training.

When testing reading with the seriously affected patient, the nurse should be sure that the grammatical forms play no part in the determination, for in this sphere as in the spoken language areas these words that make up the refinements of language are often the most difficult for the patient. Thus the nurse may print the name of an object on the paper and have the patient point to the object named, then print a common verb associated with the object and have the patient go through the indicated task. An example of this might be the name and action implied in printing the word "WATER" and then "DRINK WATER." If by showing these words without any accompanying movement or gesture indicating the act the nurse can obtain the performance, it indicates that the ability to read is retained at least in some degree. To this combination can be added the adjective "COLD" and the patient's response can be noted. If he replies correctly after drinking the water, another stage has been achieved. This example and others like it can be multiplied by many other simple acts to determine the patient's retained visual language ability.

OTHER ABILITIES. When both auditory and visual language have been attempted and the extent of the problem determined, and especially when it is found to be difficult to communicate by either the spoken or written word, the nurse should attempt to gauge the level of understanding that can be gained by gesture, facial expression, and movement imitation. This is frequently a retained language ability when the other avenues are not available. This can be best estimated by showing the patient a desired task and asking him to indicate by a shake of the head whether he can perform in a like manner. For example, the glass of water can be poured and the movement of drinking it shown by the nurse. The glass can then be handed to the patient and his movements observed or, if he shakes his head negatively indicating that he doesn't want water, his understanding of the act performed can be recognized.

In general, then, the nurse should make a determination of the language reception and performance of her patient as soon as she can. The various abilities should be probed each day, even though there was considerable difficulty in gaining any recognition the day before. The testing process itself is the first stage of therapy, for it acts as a language stimulant, and stimulation is the first requirement of all therapy.

Language Training Procedures.—The second basic principle concerns the actual training procedures in language that the nurse and others of the hospital staff can follow that will materially assist the patient in the long recovery process he faces. The importance of starting the patient off correctly cannot be stressed too much.

Where there are many hospital staff members concerned with the patient's treatment, they should all be oriented to the principles of training that are important in these first periods of recovery. In many inpatient settings this responsibility for orienting the other staff members may fall to the nurse in charge of the patient. By all pulling together, a great deal can be accomplished, especially in terms of setting the stage for an extensive training program. Where the nurse or some other single person is responsible for all or most of the handling of the patient while he is hospitalized, these basic principles must be followed consistently and carefully.

First Steps in Language Training. As a first step in training, especially for the seriously aphasic patient, the nurse should constantly probe the patient's ability to understand her spoken language. Rather than do this with sentence-long statements or questions, however, she should keep conversation at a minimum. As she handles a particular object in the room she should name it for the patient as she shows it to him. Thus, as she handles the water glass she should repeat the word "water" several times to indicate that she is naming the object in her hand. This should be done repeatedly and with several common objects, especially those with simple names and with names that can be expressed by one-syllable words.

This same process can be extended to the patient's bath. As she rubs the patient's back, the word "back" can be repeated. This type of language stimulation should not be done with a questioning voice or as though attempting to elicit the word from the patient. It is best not done in sentences. The simple repetition of the word is to be preferred to "Do you like to have your back rubbed?" or "Does it feel good as I rub your back?" These simple sentences imply a full understanding of spoken language and do not accomplish the desired result, namely the recognition by the patient that the single word being used is a symbol for the object or for the body-part being handled or referred to by the nurse.

Use of Naming Words. As has been mentioned in an earlier context the learning of language forms seems to progress from the use of naming words to other parts of speech. Naming should always be the first step. The naming process should use words that are simple, easily articulated, and clearly enunciated. Response or imitation by the patient should neither be urged nor expected. Use of language will only follow the patient's ability to integrate the cerebral cortex sufficiently to comprehend the spoken word and to produce the spoken word. It will not be achieved because it is urged by some external person or stimulus, and it does not follow from parrot-like imitation. The use of these simple naming words is intended as a stimulation of the patient on the first level of language and not as a series of stimulations that the patient may learn by repetitive drill.

One patient stimulated in this manner during an experimental training period, in which only five words were used in daily stimulation over a period of two months, did grasp the concept of symbolization but used as her first word one completely unrelated to the five words being used as direct stimulators. This same process was observed in a number of other patients where experimental conditions were not kept absolute. One patient in the latter group, although stimulated daily with such words as "water," "candy," "nose," "radio," and other common simple names, used as her first vocabulary expression the word "ladder." While this word had been used only once during the training period, it was expressed by the patient at an appropriate time as a small ladder used in the home was broken by something falling on it. The patient pointed to the wreckage and said "ladder." From these examples it is clear that the words chosen as stimulators are not in themselves important, but the fact of stimulation at the proper level seems to be. These same patients or others like them have gone for many months without either making the effort to speak or attempting it until by constant stimulation the concept of language and the integrations necessary for language, as well as the effort necessary, were all available. It is the role of the nurse or others interested in the beginning process of language training to provide this stimulation. It follows as simple logic that this stimulation should be at the lowest level, the level at which most aphasic adults return to the language process.

TRAINING IN THE PRODUCTION OF SPEECH SOUNDS. Some adult aphasics, however, need stimulation at even lower levels than the production of whole words. When the patient seems quite incapable of making purposeful sound or when sound production is attempted but seems to bear little or no relationship to the sounds used in speech, the task of training is immeasurably more difficult. To train an aphasic patient in the sounds of language requires a rather high degree of specialized skill. Wherever possible, the speech pathologist should be called upon for this part of the training process and it should not be tried by the relatively untrained nurse or others of the hospital staff.

If the nurse wishes to try such training or if it is recognized that it is going to be impossible to secure a trained speech pathologist through any source, it is advised that the nurse read one of several books on speech.[4] Any of these books will show how the different sounds of the language are formed and the mouth positions that are important in the formation. It has been found to be good practice to begin with sounds that can both be seen and be heard. This includes the lip sounds of *p* as in the word "pie," the sound *b* as in "boy," and the sound *m* as in "man." These three sounds are the simplest to teach through direct imitation.

One method suggested by Goldstein and illustrated by him in a recent book is to accompany the teaching process by some action that can represent the sound. This will bring into play the ingenuity of the nurse or instructor. For example, the sound *p* can be illustrated by the movements of the lips as smoke is expelled in a puff. The nurse should use as many teaching aids as she can, for interest can be maintained better if the stimulation is varied. She may write the letter on a blackboard in a large size, showing the position of the lips that is desired by repeating the sound a number of times. If the patient can write, he should then be asked to write the letter or copy it from the nurse's writing and to imitate the sound position, even if no sound is made. The nurse should write and say a whole series of short naming words that begin with the letter and sound *p* as "pen," "pin," "pencil," "pipe," and others, trying to use words that represent objects in the room and showing the object at the same time that the word is said. If the object is not present, she may use a picture of the object or draw the object for the patient and point to it as she says the name. At times it is wise to point to the object, picture, or drawing, then say the name, then write the name, then repeat only the sound *p,* and then indicate to the patient that he should try to say the name or the sound after the nurse as she again points to the object, the picture, or the drawing, or all three. The nurse should not be afraid of repetition; while learning itself may not be accomplished by the repetition, it may well strengthen the impression by fortifying the stimulus for the patient.

If no direct imitation or voluntary response is achieved from these processes, the nurse can try to show the sound vibrations made by producing the sound. This can be done having the patient hold

[4] R. West, L. Kennedy, and A. Carr, *Rehabilitation of Speech* (rev. ed.; New York: Harper & Bros., 1947). M. F. Berry and J. Eisenson, *The Defective in Speech* (New York: Appleton-Century-Crofts, Inc., 1947). C. Van Riper, *Speech Correction* (New York: Prentice-Hall, Inc., 1947).

his hands in front of the nurse's mouth while the puff of air is made for the *p* or having him touch the nurse's cheek or throat over the larynx while the sound *m* is made. This device of teaching the production of sound by tactual cues is widely used in work with the deaf and is found to be very helpful. One patient learned to make the sounds of the language through working first with cutouts of the different lip sounds and later with some of the others. It seemed that only by handling the rather large cardboard cutouts was it possible for him to make the connections necessary to understand the process. Another patient learned sounds and the sounding process by representing the few letters (and therefore the sounds) through a type of sign language. By forming the letter with the fingers, using the index finger and thumb of the right hand to form the semicircular top part of the letter, he was able to make the associations needed. This same process was followed for the *b* and other early sounds.

SPREAD OF RECOVERY OF OLD LEARNING. It has been found rather consistently that teaching the sounds of the language in the manner described above need not be extended to many of the individual sounds of the language. Usually the lip sounds mentioned plus the rounded vowel *o* and the full open mouth for the sound *ah* as in "arm" are enough to work with. From these the great majority of patients will get the Gestalts necessary for sound production and will go through the rest of the sounds without separate training on each sound. This follows the same process as the naming process for the word level. Only a few voluntary words need to be achieved for and with the patient directly. From that point on the patient usually begins to add other sounds and other words by himself. All training for aphasia is based upon the fact that it is not the achievement of *new* learning but rather the integrations necessary for the patient to use his old learning. This is very fortunate indeed, for if every sound and every word had to be relearned, recovery for even the best patients would be an almost endless word-relearning problem and would be even more time-consuming than is the integrative learning process.

Different patients will show this spread of learning or recovery of old learned material at very markedly different rates of speed. One patient who struggled for several months to achieve a single naming word took another two weeks to gain her second word and then began to recall her old vocabulary at a very rapid rate. Each period of training found her able to use new words, still at the same naming level, but of varying degrees of complexity. While the word "water" and the word "book" were achieved with considerable difficulty, "dictionary" and "democracy" came voluntarily soon after the first few words were learned. Re-education is a process of getting the patient started after he is capable of making the integrations and has the energy to try.

Relearning the sounds of the language follows the same rapid rate after the idea of sound production is achieved. Learning, however, goes through regular stages. The fact that sounds can be made and then new sounds self-learned or recovered from previous learning does not indicate that the rest of speech and language will follow automatically. Actually it may be just as difficult to achieve the second step as it was to achieve the first, and the nurse must be prepared for this learning by stages.

IMPORTANCE OF AN EARLY BEGINNING. During the period of hospitalization, which is usually quite limited in terms of relative time, it is not expected that the seriously affected patient will do more than possibly make a beginning at the first stage of language, whatever that stage may be in his case. What is most important, however, is that the nurse begin that first stage while the patient is hospitalized, for this beginning will make it possible for the less well-trained family member who must continue the process to take up the training. Too often the hospital staff take the viewpoint that, since the patient is to be in the hospital such a short time, it is unnecessary to begin the recovery process in terms of language training. This is precisely the wrong attitude, for it is in the very early days of recovery, when the patient can take advantage of spontaneous recovery and of the trained services of the nurse and others, that training should be started. By beginning the process the family is placed in the position of continuing an already started procedure. If the training is not begun, however, the family is in the position of having to institute something new in the daily routine, and this may be extremely difficult with many patients. By all means the training process should start as soon as the patient is capable of attending to learning even for very short periods of time.

PATIENTS WHO DO NOT PROGRESS. One other group of patients needs to be discussed in terms of early hospital training. This is the group that are not severely aphasic but that do show a considerable amount of language difficulty in either the comprehension or production of speech and do not seem to be showing very rapid spontaneous recovery, if any. For example, the patient may understand a good deal of what is said or written and be able to speak a few words if given time, but he apparently is content to stay on this rather simple language level. These patients need to be stimulated to greater efforts in speech almost as much as does the patient who appears to be totally aphasic.

Stimulation to speak and to comprehend speech means provoking the patient to try. The nurse should be sure in this process that the patient is given sufficient time to try. Too often when the aphasic patient doesn't seem to try immediately or doesn't succeed the nurse or someone else will speak for him. Unless there is some very urgent reason why an immediate response is necessary, it is better to wait for the patient to put forth the effort. If this doesn't seem to come, the nurse should restimulate. If even this is not enough, the proper procedure is to try giving short, incomplete clues as to the word expected. To illustrate, when such a patient is asked to name the common objects in the room like the "glass of water," the "radio," etc., and no response can be achieved or seems to be forthcoming, the nurse should indicate the object again and repeat the first sound in the name as *r* for "radio" or *guh* for "glass" or *puh* for "pipe." These minimal clues are frequently enough to get the patient started. It is not a good practice to begin with these verbal clues, however, for this may make the patient wait for them in the future and will not result in free and voluntary use of language. Use the verbal clues only after it is evident that the patient is not going to be able to begin the word by himself. If the verbal beginning clues are not enough and the nurse believes that the patient is becoming frustrated in his attempts to speak, she should repeat the word completely. Whatever effort the patient makes, however, should be accepted and recognized and approved verbally. For example, if the patient should succeed in making the first sound of a word and then lapse into silence, the nurse should complete the word for him and approve his effort rather than urge him to try to complete it alone. His abortive effort is apparently as far as he can take it at that time, and the same effects will be found from this urging process as were noted earlier when patients were given every assistance because the effort was completely aborted. Constant approval of any and every effort should be a standing rule. Urging or pressuring the patient to continue to try after he has shown an inability to perform should never be a part of the training process. The nurse can secure a greater effort and a continuing one by repeating the question or shifting to another; psychologically this will accomplish much more.

ACCEPTANCE OF POOR ARTICULATION.   One important generalization must be remembered regarding the speech efforts of the aphasic patient. The problem is one of an inability to integrate the cortical processes for the complex task of comprehending or producing language. As language is recovered, there will be noted very often an inability or a tendency to articulate the new words rather badly. Thus a patient attempting to say "ball" may produce a word like "baw" or "paw." While it would seem proper to correct these poor articulatory attempts, this should not be done. In the first place, attempted correction will imply criticism of the effort, and the patient needs all the acceptance and approval he can get. In the second place the more important problem is the symbolic act of producing a word that can be understood as a satisfactory verbalization; by producing the approximate word or the correct word poorly articulated, the basic problem has been overcome. Speech or good articulation is important, but for the aphasic patient it must be secondary to the act of using propositional language. Correction of poor speech can be done at any time after language is achieved and should not be a part of the early training process.

Summary

To summarize very briefly the inpatient phase of recovery from brain injury and the role of the hospital staff in the recovery process, it is important to re-emphasize the need for beginning therapy while the patient is in the very early stages of recovery. Experience has shown that patients whose training has started in these early convalescent days have much the better chance of eventually achieving maximal recovery. The entire hospital staff is responsible for this therapy, the doctor, nurse, physiotherapist, occupational therapist, social worker, psychologist, and speech therapist. Usually it is recognized that the major burden will fall upon the nurse, and the discussion has centered upon her role since it epitomizes the role of most of the others.

First, there must be recognition of the common expected behavioral aberrations. From recognition must come a better handling of these same problems. Lack of initiative, impulsive behavior, frustration reaction patterns, so-called catastrophic reactions, need for planned rest and stimulation periods, tendency toward concreteness and away from the abstract, egocentricity, and lack of interest in the rest of the world, plus early euphoria, are all tendencies which the nurse and the others of the hospital staff must train themselves to deal with competently. Finally, some immediate suggestions for language training have been offered. These have covered quite briefly an investigation of the type and degree of aphasia and some of the more general considerations in starting the actual training process. The importance of early training of the brain-injured patient cannot be stressed too much. It is the pathway established by the hospital staff that may well be the deciding factor for many patients between a partial recovery on the one hand and a return to a useful life on the other.

Chapter 11

ASSOCIATED THERAPIES AND THERAPISTS: II. SECONDARY STAGE OF RECOVERY

On discharge from the hospital it can be assumed that the aphasic patient has passed through the initial stage of recovery, where the emphasis has been properly placed upon his physical and medical needs. While he is still in need of considerable physical care and medical treatment, his condition as he returns to the home should warrant a shift of emphasis to psychological and language recovery. The patient should no longer be considered as physically ill, but rather as suffering from a language handicap which may be complicated by psychological and physical impairment. He faces the imposing task of readjustment and rehabilitation structured by his difficulty in communication, his paralysis, and what may be considered as his new patterns of reaction to self and to the world. In terms used by some present-day investigators, he may be described as possessing the potential for many if not all the personality strengths and weaknesses that were his prior to his trauma, but biologically his intelligence factors are different and he must develop new approaches to a new existence. This is the task facing the people in his immediate environment, his family and sometimes his friends. They must assist him in recovery—not in becoming the individual that he was before, but in re-establishing his ability to utilize his potentials in language, in physique, and in psyche.

Objectives in Home Care

The primary stage of this recovery was spent in the hospital where he had the ministrations of his physicians, nurses, and others of the professional staff. Now he passes into the hands of his well-meaning, but usually quite untrained, family circle. In the past this has meant in almost every case that the aphasic patient would receive a maximum of continued physical care and a minimum of language re-education and psychological assistance. The results have been about as one would expect. Physically these patients have prospered and as invalids have enjoyed comparatively long but inactive lives.

Psychologically and in language, however, the progression has been almost nil. Usefulness—the resumption of a relatively normal life or the re-establishment of a responsible place in society—has rarely been achieved. It is the attempt to reopen this door to recovery that the present volume strives for, and training by the family is one of the primary methods available and necessary.

It is recognized that some patients, rather than returning to the home, spend a considerable period of time in nursing homes or convalescent centers. The rehabilitation problems in these secondary homes are not unlike the problems faced in the patient's own home, and for that reason the second stage of recovery will be treated as a unit.

Aphasia therapists, social workers, nurses, or physicians who have attempted to assist families in their efforts to participate in the therapeusis of aphasic patients have always been faced by the difficult problem of orienting and training the families to assume the role of therapists. In the following pages some of the areas in which the families can be maximally useful will be discussed. Some of the problems faced by the aphasia patient during his early recovery period will be shown, and some suggestions will be made for overcoming these problems. These remarks are directed to the families, per se, although it is recognized that they will serve their best function if they are relayed to the families by someone trained in therapy and re-education. The professional consultant will recognize the impossibility of applying any set, prearranged series of lessons to the individual aphasic patient. Each such patient must be approached individually with a flexible program designed to meet his needs; no over-all program can be devised to meet all problems. The suggestions made can therefore be best used as suggestive techniques that may apply in one form or another to many types of patients.

The Area of Physical Care

Most aphasic patients upon return to their homes are still in need of considerable physical care. In every instance they should be under the surveillance of a physician acquainted with their difficulty. This means more than having handy the name of a physician to whom the family can refer in time of need. Rather, one physician, well acquainted with the patient and with the family, who can regularly advise the family concerning the physical and medical problems involved is a better solution. Questions about medication for an existing or continuing medical condition; questions concerning diet; questions concerning physiotherapy and the need for massage, diathermy, or exercise; questions concerning prostheses for paralyzed extremities; and questions about general guidance and assistance of the patient should always be referred to the attending physician. Even when the condition is apparent and the assistance necessary seems to be self-evident, the family should seek and follow the physician's advice. As the physical problems appear to become static and treatment for the patient has become stabilized, the doctor should be called upon for routine examinations several times during the year. New medication is constantly being discovered, new theories concerning treatment are being proved in the laboratories, new prosthetic devices are always being tested, and new surgical procedures are being devised. The families can hope to keep abreast of these new and progressive methods only by keeping in constant touch with their physician.

Convulsive Seizures.—The doctor will recognize the tendency toward convulsive seizures and when indicated will prescribe the proper medication. Home remedies and patent medicines should never be used. They are worse than a poor choice; they may do actual harm. The condition itself requires only the most careful medical guidance. Improper medication may lead to the most devastating effects. The family should always contact their physician whenever the patient indicates that he is dizzy, or when he faints or shows other signs of losing consciousness. The effects of these convulsions or convulsive-like behavior can often be controlled by proper medication. The benefits that will derive from following this suggestion will far offset any temporary inconvenience caused by calling the physician. This is one problem that the family should not under any circumstances attempt to handle alone.

Paralysis.—Most prominent among the physical defects seen in the brain-injured patient is the common paralysis of the extremities of one side of the body, especially the right hand and leg, but sometimes also affecting the right side of the face. This is called a hemiplegia, which means a half-paralysis—one-half of the body is paralyzed. Sometimes this paralysis is only partial, and the arm may be affected without the leg's suffering at all. At other times, but not as commonly, the leg and not the arm is affected. These complete or partial losses of function do decrease in severity—the arm or the leg may regain its function either completely or partly. The leg function usually recovers more quickly and more completely than the arm. Physiotherapy, planned exercise, heat treatments, and hydrotherapy may be important in this recovery process, and the family should seek the guidance of their physician in planning this phase of care for the patient. Restoration of function in a paralyzed arm or leg takes a long time. Treatment should be started as soon as possible. Where professional physiotherapy cannot be obtained, the physician can often advise the family about home treatment for the condition.

Headaches.—In some brain-injured patients headaches are common. Usually these headaches will not respond to ordinary home treatment and the doctor should again be sought out for possible helpful medication. It is wise to seek such help, for constant headaches may be a symptom of remaining irritation in the brain, and this may need careful study by the doctor in order to find a means of correcting the condition. The persistent headaches are also very bad psychologically. Patients become irritable and unable to participate in planned training procedures if they are beset by constant, or even intermittent, severe headaches. New drugs are being developed, fortunately, that may assist many patients in overcoming these persistent, irritating symptoms, and these should be used under the doctor's guidance.

Defective Vision.—Many aphasic patients complain of difficulty in vision. In some this may be directly due to their brain damage. If the patient cannot read (and most aphasic patients have difficulty in reading), they often assume that the difficulty lies in their ability to see. It is wise to check vision whenever it is a problem to the patient. Frequently it will not be found to be an actual visual acuity defect, but ruling out the possibility is important. A considerable amount of time can be wasted in training if a visual acuity defect is present but not recognized. Some patients may have a different type of visual problem that affects their ability to read. This fairly common defect does not concern the usual eye weakness that is seen in many people and is correctable by glasses, but a special type of visual problem. This type is called a *visual field defect*—that is certain parts of both the right and left eye are affected and objects off to the far right (or left) cannot be seen at all. *Visual field* is the term used to describe the whole span of vision that everyone has —the distance to the right or left that can be visualized without turning the head. Just as one half of the body may be paralyzed as described earlier, one half of the field of vision may be blacked out. When the patient complains that he cannot see, his vision can be checked by moving objects that he says are out of his range of vision over in front of him. If he then can see them, he probably has this visual field problem and should be studied by an eye doctor. The family physician should be consulted about this. No remedy may exist for the condition, but if the family understands the problem they can then assist the patient by being sure that all objects that he is attempting to see are placed within his range of vision. The family and the patient should know that visual problems of this type are not progressive and do not mean that anything further is likely to happen that will make the vision worse. It is merely a part of the total problem of the brain-injured patient and must be dealt with practically and objectively. As soon as the patient can understand such problems and accept them for their true value, they should be explained to him so that he may learn to adjust to them.

Diet and Exercise.—Other physical problems occur in many aphasic patients. With some, diet is very important, and the physician should be consulted about this during the early days at home. Since most aphasic brain-injured patients are forced to be inactive, and if paralyzed are unable to exercise properly, they need careful dietary study. Prepared diets that will provide the necessary food values without increase in weight are of extreme importance and should be followed quite rigorously. Along with proper food intake, the family should seek guidance as to the amount and type of exercise that the patient should have. It was unfortunately a common bit of advice in the past that the brain-injured patient should rest and not be active in any way for a considerable period of time after his return home. This is no longer considered as good general advice. The doctor is in the best position to know how much and what kind of exercise is advisable for the patient.

Early attempts at walking even for the paralyzed patient are strongly advised. The sooner the patient can master some self-controlled locomotion, the more rapidly can he develop comparative independence. Language stimulation is also greatly improved, since opportunities for external contacts are increased by the extended environment possible through walking. In addition, the psychological advantages are evident. As the patient regains function in his extremities and independence through his recovery of motion, confidence can be gained and anxieties and frustrations concerning the future may be less evident. As will be seen in a later section, activity is an important part of the total therapeutic process. Walking, and the general exercise it entails, is a very essential part of the activity possible for the patient.

In closing this section on physical care it should be restated that the advice of the physician should be sought for all the physical and medical care needed by the patient. His advice should be followed rigorously. It is better to ask too many questions about physical care than too few. It is vital to the whole recovery program that the patient be as free of physical disability as possible. Home remedies and old family treatments have no place in a recovery program for the brain-injured patient. Only the most competent medical care should be sought and followed by the family.

Psychological Considerations

Equally important in the recovery process is the psychological understanding and care of the aphasic patient. For the most part the patient will be seen to be the same person he was before his illness, but there will be observed in most patients a whole series of new behavior patterns. These may have the effect of making the family think that the patient is different; that he is more irritable, less interested in the family or in other people, and quite content to sit for hours doing nothing. These frequently observed bits of behavior and the many others discussed in earlier chapters (see especially Chapter 3) may be seen for the first time as the patient comes home. Some of these behavior mechanisms are believed to be the direct result of the brain injury itself. For example, the short attention-span and the apparent difficulty in concentration that so many brain-injured patients show are apparently due to the inability of the patient to integrate his thought processes and keep them trained on the problem at hand. In part this may be best understood as being what one investigator has described as loss in the area of biological intelligence.[1] This, simply expressed, means loss of the ability to block out of the mind emotional attitudes and other internalized feelings while attempting to pay conscious attention to the task at hand. Such direct results of brain injury tend to make the patient seem flighty and wandering in his attention, whereas they actually indicate that his brain is going through a process of reintegration and needs outside assistance to return to the task presented to it.

Falling into this category of supposed direct psychological results of brain injury, as previously noted, is the loss of memory which is so frequently seen (see also pages 19 to 35). This is especially noticeable in the brain-injured patient during the early recuperative

---

[1] Ward C. Halstead, *Brain and Intelligence* (Chicago: University of Chicago Press, 1948).

period, but may last well into the secondary stages as well. New memories or very recent events are especially difficult for the average patient. One patient for example had extreme difficulty in recalling such recent events as the kind of food he had eaten for breakfast just an hour previously. Two days later, however, when asked what he had eaten on that day he was able to name three of the four items on the breakfast menu. It is often seen in the area of recall that old personal memories are quite intact, while events that happened in the recent past are sometimes confused and very recent happenings are quite difficult to recall. Fortunately, most patients seem to overcome this aspect of their general problem with the passage of time. The writer feels that the stimulation of recall through therapy plays a fairly important role in the recovery of memory.

A loss or disturbance of the ability to abstract is another extremely common psychological disturbance after brain injury (see also page 24). One writer offers considerable data to show that disruption of the ability to abstract appears consistently as a sign of brain injury.[2] Others hold that there is likely to be such a disturbance, but that it does not always appear and that when it does it is more a matter of degree than an absolute loss.[3] One thing that is agreed upon by almost all investigators is that such disturbances of thought do appear very frequently and that in many such patients they appear to the degree that only the most concrete stimuli can be understood. To illustrate the way in which this disability appears, consider the patient who when shown an inverted V could only understand it as the gable of a house. When two separate lines were shown to him in the manner of an equals sign in a simple arithmetic problem, he failed to see the relationship, since the sign represented an abstraction he was unable to comprehend and was not readily translatable into a concrete form as was the inverted V. Another patient when shown a pipe and asked what it was for, would reply "Smoke," but when the pipe was not shown and the question was asked, "What do you do with a pipe?" he could not visualize the subject of the question and could not respond. Still another patient, previously extremely interested in baseball, could not discuss the merits of the local team, became quite disinterested in a verbal discussion of the game being played and apparently could not follow references to the

---

[2] Kurt Goldstein, *Language and Language Disturbances* (New York: Grune & Stratton, Inc., 1948).

[3] Jon Eisenson, "Aphasics: Observations and Tentative Conclusions," *Journal of Speech Disorders*, XII (September, 1947), 291–92. Robert Leepert, "Cognitive and Symbolic Processes," chapter in unpublished manuscript, University of Oregon, 1949.

game that were made by the therapist. When his television set was turned on, however, he could understand what was said to him about the game and could follow rather complicated references to the players and the positions they occupied on the team.

Objectivity in Training.—Recognition of these facts about the thought processes of the aphasic patient makes it important that all discussion and training be very objective and very real. Everything discussed with the patient should be present, visible, and even touchable if necessary. The family should take care that they do not introduce material that was of pretraumatic interest to the patient if this material necessitates an abstract attitude in the patient for his consideration of it. For example, if the subject being discussed is food, the food should be present. What was eaten for breakfast or what the patient would like to have for lunch may be far too abstract a thought for him to handle. While different patients vary in the degree of their loss of ability to abstract and their consequent need to have everything very concrete, it is wise to assume that a more or less absolute concreteness of thought exists until the family can determine the actual degree of abstracting ability possessed by the patient. This is especially true of markedly aphasic patients. All stimuli and all material used in training should be very real and very objective; otherwise there may be a great delay in learning.

Allowance for Inability to Utilize Retained Intellect.—Still another area of psychological disturbance believed due directly to brain damage concerns what is called here the ability to utilize the retained intellect. This is best observed in a whole series of events which represent common reactions to intellectual problems as seen in both test and real situations as performed by many brain-injured patients. The most frequently seen of these mechanisms are (a) poor ability to organize material, (b) poor use of judgment, (c) inability to shift easily from one situation to another, (d) real difficulty in adjusting to new situations when the shift has been made, (e) inability to correct responses made even though they are known to be incorrect, and (f) apparent generalized loss of what is commonly called intelligence. These different psychological signs do not appear in every patient. To most people these signs may not appear to be present unless they are demonstrated, and they may appear very overtly at some times when they had previously not been noticed. When they do appear, and when they are recognized, they should be accepted as concomitants of brain injury and not as wilful behavior. As has been indicated in an earlier context (see Chapter 6), many of these signs disappear with therapy. The following excerpt from a case history illustrates the effect of these factors on one of the patients studied by the author:

The patient was a forty-two-year-old married white male. He was the father of three teen-age children. His wife was ill with a debilitating heart condition which had invalidized her for many years. At the time of the patient's discharge from the hospital, the wife was at home but confined to her bed. After a two-month hospitalization for a brain injury suffered in an automobile accident the patient was discharged to his home. The most prominent sign of his disability was a severe expressive aphasia.

In planning therapy it was necessary for the oldest child to act as the primary therapist. During the early home convalescence every decision necessary in the home was referred to the patient for his concurrence. This even extended to the area of therapy. A whole series of events followed this procedure. A daily schedule was developed but was found to be quite impractical after only a few days' trial. The time estimated for the performance of the many home duties as well as the sequence that had been determined for their performance had been quite unrealistic. (Note the poor organizing and the use of poor judgment.) When taxed with this failure by the eldest child, the patient seemed to study the outlined plan but although not suffering from difficulty in reading, he seemed quite incapable of understanding what was wrong. (Note here the inability to abstract and the inability to correct errors which he had made and that he knew were errors.) The children assisted the father in his efforts at self-recovery of writing and speaking, but they soon noted that when he became frustrated he would not be able to skip the obstacle and go on to something else, but would continue to try, even though unsuccessful, to conquer that one presenting error. When he was urged to shift to another problem he would find it extremely difficult to accommodate himself to the new situation. Frustration would appear much more rapidly, and he would soon cease working altogether. (Note the difficulty in shifting and the increased frustration when faced by the new situation in the training process.) Recognizing after a time that there was little change in her father, the eldest child called on the family doctor, who secured the services of an aphasia therapist to direct and guide the recovery program.

The importance of these intellectualizing factors on therapy cannot be stressed too strongly. The best of effort and the most well-meaning assistance that does not take them into consideration will only produce increased frustration and anxiety in the patient and will block the recovery rather than assist it.

Handling the Problem of Anxiety.—During the early phases of recovery it has already been noted that many aphasic adults show a distinct attitude of euphoria. That is, they appear to be quite happy and unconcerned about their condition. Coupled with this feeling of well-being in many brain-injured patients are the additional psychological signs of constriction of interest to self and the immediate environment and marked egocentricity. When euphoria is present, the patient rarely seems anxious about anything, including his past ability, his future economic status, his illness and operation, and everything else. As time goes on, however, most patients learn to become anxious and concerned.

In observing many aphasic patients as they were reintroduced to their families and their friends for the first time, it became apparent that they developed these attitudes of despair and depression in almost direct relation to the anxiety and concern of the people around them. Thus, when the wife or mother of a patient became emotional about his condition, talked to the patient about the difficult time they would have from then on, related the general and very real problems of life that the family faced and the patient's inability to be of help, made consistent and repeated references to the patient's previous ability to talk or to earn or even to play various games, and expressed in other ways their own feelings of insecurity to the patient, then the patient began to worry. Marked anxieties were established and even with intense therapy thereafter, the so-called "ghost of the past" was always present and had its inevitable bad effect upon therapy. Establishing future goals is always difficult with the aphasic patient, but if approached slowly and realistically they can be of great value in motivating the patient to continued effort. When, however, they are presented as impossible attainments that require future planning (something that few brain-injured patients can do), they invariably produce anxiety and deep concern and a marked feeling of futility in the patient.

Most brain-injured patients will develop anxiety about their condition and about their improvement as they go along in therapy. If they are succeeding in overcoming some of the defect, they usually are able to handle this anxiety quite well. The family must be very careful not to extend this attitude or not to produce anxiety where it doesn't already exist. If the family or members of the group immediately around the patient find that they cannot control their own feelings about the patient and his future, they should, first, try to avoid showing this lack of control to the patient and, second, stay away from the patient as much as possible. For the aphasic patient, the only method that has been found generally useful in allaying anxiety is the day-by-day proof that comes from effort and success. Consequently the attitude of the therapist and the family must be one of constant encouragement. Therapy must be planned that will produce success. While it is necessary in order to secure a good learning situation to stimulate the patient with problems that he must solve and obstacles that he must overcome which may be difficult for him, yet every effort toward solution of those problems must be praised and further effort secured through the approbation. Criticism or an attitude of implying that the patient could do much better or one that suggests that he has failed and must therefore try again will usually result in refusal and rejection if continued. This immediate refusal may not appear to be too serious, but if it is continued deep-seated anxieties may develop in the patient, and then therapy may be extremely difficult.

Avoiding a Show of Emotion.—In the same way the family must learn to hide their feelings of deep emotion, of oversentimentalizing about the patient. The problem that the patient shows can be overcome only with a very real and objective attitude. In some families this may mean that the one person closest to the patient may be the wrong person to direct the training program. An illustration of this is seen in the following case history:

This patient was a man of some sixty years who had spent an active and useful life as a merchant in another country and then had emigrated to America during a period of stress in his native land. He had faced this readjustment well, as had his wife and one child. In this country he had worked usefully and with fair success for some eight years, mastering at his advanced age a new language and a new mode of life. His wife had retained a firm conviction of his ability to earn a satisfactory living and to make a new home.

Suffering a cerebral accident, he was left unparalyzed but severely aphasic. He then understood no English and only a bare minimum of his native tongue. Without initial training as described in previous chapters of the present book, he withdrew into a protective shell. His contacts with the world were limited to his wife, his daughter, and his son-in-law. The latter two attempted to pierce this armor of defense, but, since they lived away from the parental home, their influence was partial and intermittent. The wife became depressed and anxious, not particularly about the economic future, for there was enough money for the couple to live comfortably if not luxuriously, but about the condition of her husband. She succeeded even in the early posttraumatic period in transmitting her insecurity and anxiety to the patient. Every spontaneous effort he made was negated by her instant comparison with his previous ability. His behavior became more and more withdrawn. He became in effect exactly what his wife believed him to be, an ineffectual, withdrawn man. The world had passed him by, and he was awaiting with his wife an inevitable surcease from his difficulties.

As long as the wife remained the prime mover in the family, this condition continued. The daughter and her husband attempted to be helpful at first, but they found the atmosphere at home to be so depressing that their visits became further and further apart and the patient and his wife became more and more secluded.

This condition obtained until the daughter, spurred by an accidental reading of a popular journal describing work with aphasic patients during the recent war, stimulated the patient to seek outside assistance. After several months of therapy it was possible to isolate the different aspects of the aphasic problem. It was found that the patient could understand and work rather well in his first learned language. Therapy was provided in that language, and at the same time supportive psychotherapy was suggested for the wife. By combining this dual program it was possible to achieve a fair degree of recovery. For over six months, however, it was necessary to exclude the wife from the therapeusis, and most of the actual training was accomplished despite her continuous attitude of hopelessness, which seemed all too well to succeed in negating the positive steps taken by the daughter and the therapist.

To be successful in rehabilitating the aphasic patient, the family must attain an objective, unemotional attitude toward the problem. Case histories can be shown of effects, equally as devastating as in the above case, when the family is overemotional in sympathizing with the physical ailments. A practical, objective attitude, however, one that faces the reality of the task, but that also recognizes the value of training and work, can achieve minor miracles in many seemingly hopeless cases.

Preparing the Family for Rehabilitation of the Patient

Another principle, one that seems self-evident but that experience shows is easily overlooked, deals with the preparation of the family to undertake the task of rehabilitation. One of the fundamental questions posed in family training for aphasia concerns the possibility of securing assistance. In most communities today, and the influence is spreading, there are speech correctionists. In many states there are growing services offered by state or municipal educational units in the areas of speech and psychology. Through our universities and colleges these specialists are securing training in understanding some of the basic principles regarding recovery from aphasic disturbances. Most often a letter to the state university or to the local college or to the state department of education will secure information concerning the possibilities of obtaining such trained assistance. A letter to the American Speech and Hearing Association through Dr. George A. Kopp, its secretary at Wayne University, Detroit, Michigan, will bring information concerning the qualified speech pathologists in any locality in the United States. This help may not be available for every aphasic patient, but advice and guidance for the family can be obtained in most cases. While this may not be completely satisfactory, it will offer the kind of support in most cases that will start the family off on the road to recovery, even though all the actual training and care remain in their hands. In one case where the patient lived in Mexico, the patient's wife was able to secure the assistance of a very competent teacher who through the application of good teaching principles, plus some correspondence with the author, was able to be of marked assistance to the family and the patient.

The family also should take advantage of all the guidance and suggestion that they can get from their physician or from the sources that he may suggest. If the hospital has been instrumental in establishing the kind of beginning therapy suggested earlier, the family should seek out each member of the hospital staff who has been in contact with the patient and carry on the different functions for the patient that the different specialists have instituted. Where this was not the beginning course and the only hospital contacts the patient had were with the nursing and medical staffs of the hospital, these people should be sought out and as complete a picture as possible of the patient's behavior and condition while hospitalized should be obtained. In the main all that is suggested here is that the family should attempt to carry on what has already been started. When, however, no assistance in this direction has been obtained or is possible after the early convalescent stage, the family should still seek the assistance of their physician for the guidance they need in caring for the physical side of the patient's problem. Perhaps he will be able to suggest other sources of assistance as well.

Each family must study its particular problem. The members must notice the differences between the patient's behavior after his injury and before. They should not expect spontaneous return to the personality and intelligence of the pretraumatic state—changes, whatever they may be, will come about only by careful work and training. They should be understood as being caused by alteration in the nervous system. In the process of recovery the patient regains the ability to integrate his brain functions, and he must be given every possible assistance. Most important of all. the family must remember that assistance does not mean constant help—oversolicitous attention, catering to whims, or too much sympathy. It means reducing anxiety by not being anxious; reducing frustration and irritation by shifting stimulus material and subject matter; taking advantage of euphoria when it is present by establishing a regime in which the patient tries to help himself; and understanding the patient and his needs rather than performing for him. By studying the common behavioral signs, understanding them in terms of the behavior of the individual patient being cared for, and being helpful when help is needed, a great deal can be accomplished.

The Area of Language Care and Re-education

Language training to overcome the patient's difficulty in communication is the third big sphere of activity, in addition to physical and psychological care, in which the family must orient itself. While this may appear to be an overwhelming task, a good deal can be accomplished if certain basic principles of communication and training are kept in mind. It is not expected that the family will become trained professional teachers or therapists, but there is so much that can be done by every family that there is no need to permit the patient to become a permanent invalid and dependent for the rest of his life. These suggestions of course will not cover every emergency. They will be general, and only a part of them may apply to any one patient, but they can be helpful for the most part with almost any patient. They should be used as they are presented if they seem appropriate; if not, they should be modified to fit the need of the particular problem.

Evaluation of Expressive Ability.—The first task is to evaluate the patient's ability to use words to express ideas. This can be done very simply by observation. How does he communicate his needs? Does he use words when he wants something, or does he point? If he uses words, are they appropriate to what he wants? For instance, if he wants a glass of water, does he say "water" or does he merely point to the glass? Or if he attempts to speak the word as he points, does he say the expected word or some other word or phrase?

Most aphasic adults have automatic words or phrases that they use whenever they attempt language. Sometimes these automatisms are quite complex. One patient, whenever he attempted speech, would say "County jail—murder—Phoenix" rapidly and with inflection while pointing to the object he wanted. This was evidently inappropriate and easily recognized as such, but another patient would preface every attempt with "I say." At first it was believed that this was the beginning of a sentence and would be followed by a statement, but the rest of the speech did not follow the phrase, and it was then recognized as an automatic verbalization and quite unrelated to communication. One should observe, then, the patient's ability to express himself. If he has some words at his command, he should have every possible opportunity to use them. Questions can be framed that will elicit the words that he can produce. This will give him encouragement and will fortify his later efforts at other words.

Evaluation of Understanding.—At the same time one should make a rough evaluation of the patient's ability to understand language. Does he follow remarks addressed to him? This is best seen in actions that he performs and usually is not sufficiently tested if he merely nods his head in response to a question. His understanding of speech should be gauged by his behavior. For example, if one says "Do you want a glass of water?" and he responds by reaching for the glass held out to him, it does not mean that he has understood the spoken question. Questions should be framed so that the answers will provide a measure of the patient's ability to understand words without other clues. For example, he may be asked to turn on a radio or to point at a simple object within the room, without any other indication of the radio or other object. He should be tested out in this way many times, with long and short sentences and long and short words. One patient appeared to follow many radio programs, asking by motions that certain programs be turned on and rejecting other programs when they were substituted, yet it was evident from her behavior that it was not the context of the program that was being selected since by every observation she did not understand the spoken voice. Still another patient always requested the morning paper and spent a considerable time going through it page by page, yet by every test tried he could not understand the printed word in any form. Do not judge understanding by verbal language since these patients are often totally incapable of verbal communication. Do not judge understanding by generalized behavior as described above. Do make your judgments by repeated observations of simple behavior in response to directed questions or tasks.

Stimulation of Understanding.—In the beginning, after determination of the patient's ability to understand, one should plan to spend several short periods each day in direct stimulation of the patient. The simplest course to follow is to take a seat near the patient when he is rested and willing to work and to begin by pointing to an object in the room that has a common name and saying it aloud, then indicating without words, if possible, that the patient should try the same name. Imitation of the naming used is not important. It is often better to select a few common objects and name them several times as they are indicated, without urging the patient to respond in any way. The series of names is repeated several times. After it is evident that the patient hears some one name, one should try eliciting a response from him by merely pointing to the article in question or by holding it up. For example, one may arrange a glass of water, a book, a pencil, and a pipe on a convenient table; then pick up the glass and say the word "water"; after replacing it, pick up a pencil and say "pencil—pencil—pencil," doing the same with the book and the pipe, repeating each name several times. One may then repeat the whole series, altering the order each time.

After this procedure has been followed several times, one may pick up the object and point to the patient, indicating that he should try. If he succeeds in saying anything, one should smile and agree with him, not expecting accuracy of enunciation or completeness of expression. If he does not succeed, the word should be repeated several times, without asking the patient to imitate it. One should continue by picking up the next object and repeating the same process, rewarding every effort and giving the patient all the time he needs to try, whether he succeeds or not. If he tries and seems to be frustrated in his attempts, one should either go directly to the next object or repeat the name the patient is trying to get. This type of exercise may have to be repeated several times a day and for many days, keeping the stimulus articles the same. If no success can be obtained by word repetition in this way, adding written clues may be tried. As the object is pointed out and the name repeated, one should print the name on a piece of paper while saying it. If necessary, one may accompany each showing of the object with an appropriate use of it, showing the patient that the water is for drinking, the book for reading, the pencil for writing, the pipe for smoking, etc. Other language should be kept at a minimum during these beginning exercises. Actually, it is helpful to refrain from other talking during these periods.

During the rest of the day, whenever the opportunity presents itself, these same articles should be referred to by their single-word names. At mealtime one may indicate the glass of water and say "water." In writing a letter in the patient's presence, using a pencil. one may hold it up and say "pencil," etc. These informal situations should not be made tiresome by going out of the way to find opportunities to use the words, but they should be used whenever the opportunity presents itself.

This process of naming must be remembered as the first stage of training. Language is learned in most instances by single words in four stages. The first is naming—the use of common nouns. The second is action—the use of verbs. The third is modifications of the noun—the use of adjectives. The fourth is modification of the verb—the use of adverbs. The second stage should not be attempted until the patient can respond fairly easily to the first. The third and fourth stages follow the others in regular order. There is no basic law of learning involved in this order. It has merely been observed that this is the simplest order for patients to follow in regaining language. It may take many months before the patient is able to add words by himself at any of the stages. It is this spontaneous addition of words that indicates the patient's ability to function at that level in a normal way. Usually it is wise to continue a particular stage until the patient does make some of his own additions to his vocabulary.

An important consideration is the grammatical problem. One should not be concerned about the little grammatical words—the prepositions, articles, conjunctions, etc. Patients suffering from aphasia invariably have difficulty in adding grammar to language, and it is only at a very late stage of training that these words can be added. A typical procedure is to begin with the one-word sentence—the name or noun—following this with the pronouns, especially the personal pronouns. After the patient indicates his ability to use a fair number of nouns—that is, to name a number of objects voluntarily with little urging or delay—one should shift to the two-word sentence, the noun plus verb. The verbs "to be" and "to have" should be avoided, as these are usually very difficult for any aphasic patient. Simple action verbs that can be demonstrated are best, for example, "pencil write," "water drink," "book read," "ball throw," "food eat," and others at this level. When some two-word sentences are produced, one may change to the simple pronoun forms. "I drink water" and "You read paper" are examples. Adjectives should be added after some of these sentences are used. "He drinks cold water," "I sit down fast," "The water is cold." After the patient has reached this level, it is usually found that he will add many new sentences himself.

One of the things the family therapist must be careful of is the tendency to accept a minimal effort as being a satisfactory goal. If the patient has not talked at all for a considerable period and the teaching process has become quite burdensome until finally single naming-words are attained, there is a tendency to consider that a satisfactory level of achievement. If the family so considers it, the patient will be sure to accept it. If the patient can succeed in mastering single names and using them purposively, there is no reason to believe that he cannot go on to higher levels of communication.

In the early stages of training there is a very definite advantage to using the same stimulus material over and over. During later stages, however, the material should be shifted constantly as the patient exhibits continuous frustration or rejection of the training effort.

Reading and Writing.—Reading can usually be added during a fairly early stage of training. Even simple word recognition like having the patient pick words out of the headlines of newspapers is helpful. He should copy the words that he knows, read them aloud, and then try to use them in talking after he has read them. For more intense work in reading, a beginning book from a local school or library is useful. The instructions given in the book for the order of presentation should be followed, but one should not expect the same type of reading changes that are seen in the child learning to read. For additional help in this area, Dolch's manual on remedial reading techniques [4] and Fernald's excellent and suggestive book on all school subjects [5] may be found extremely helpful. Usually reading aloud follows the progress made in speaking aloud. Reading silently often follows oral reading but just as often seems to be self-taught by constant exposure and effort on the patient's part.

A common practice is to begin writing exercises soon after the first voluntary words are spoken. If books make instruction easier, try Freeman's practice books [6] when the patient does not show a paralysis of the arm that he formerly used for writing and Gardner's manual for left-handed writing [7] if the patient is paralyzed. Many patients, however, can learn to write by themselves by first learning to copy from printed material. At the beginning it has been found to be extremely important to advise the patient to write very large. Sometimes the letters should be formed as large as four or five

[4] E. W. Dolch, *A Manual for Remedial Reading* (Champaign, Ill.: The Garrard Press, 1945).

[5] G. M. Fernald, *Remedial Techniques in Basic School Subjects* (New York: McGraw-Hill Book Co., Inc., 1943).

[6] F. N. Freeman, *Correlated Handwriting: Practice Books 1, 2, and 3* (Columbus, O.: Zaner-Bloser Co., 1931).

[7] Warren Gardner, *Left-Handed Writing* (Danville, Ill.: Interstate Press, 1945).

inches, with only a few words to a page. Some patients have had to begin the writing process on blackboards, using chalk and writing six- or seven-inch letters before they could master the movements necessary. Ordinarily printing is learned easier than cursive writing. The change to ordinary script can be made as soon as the patient seems able to make the coordinating movements necessary.

The newspaper, with its large headlines, usually makes good stimulus material for both reading and writing. Self-help should be encouraged as much as possible. A table may be set up and the patient may be told to copy from the newspaper while he is alone. In general, the patient should be encouraged to do as much work as he can while alone. This usually requires a considerable amount of urging and encouragement, but it has been noted that many patients seem to progress best when they try to help themselves in reading and writing while no one else is around. This self-effort should be encouraged after some success has been obtained by the patient in working with family members, *but it should not be instituted at the very beginning.*

In both reading and writing it has been found easiest to work with large printed material rather than small book-sized print. One should not be concerned with omitted words or occasional lapses in copying. Specific correction of articulation of poorly enunciated words should not be attempted until language is fairly well developed. It is best to work for language first and accuracy last in all forms— speaking, reading, and writing.

The inadequacy of these paragraphs as a complete course of training for the aphasic adult is recognized. They are of course not intended to be such a complete course. Actually the family must be ingenious in devising new methods and using new stimulations that possibly have never been tried before. No text can be complete for every patient. The sections on training for the aphasia therapist in later chapters may be helpful in suggesting new things to try for particular parts of the language disorder. The books suggested throughout the chapter can be obtained from any bookstore. One should not hesitate to try new things, for stimulating the patient in many ways is good for him.

Summary

Language recovery, it must be remembered, is far, far more than the number of words a patient can use, the ability to read by sight recognition when stimulated, the ability to write what is suggested, or any of the other individual communication skills that have been discussed. It includes and is based upon the patient's ability to form useful concepts and to use them freely without stimulation. The immediate goals of training should never be complicated by attempts either to improve the articulation of the patient or to extend his vocabulary. Articulatory skill can be trained at a much later date when the patient can attend to the polishing of speech which is present. Vocabulary will develop within the patient by recall of previously learned words after the ability to gain and hold concepts has been recovered. New learning is not involved. The family must be able to keep under control the abnormal psychological factors which impede recovery. They must be able to view the patient and his problem objectively and not sentimentally. They must be able to subjugate their own needs for speech and to keep their language at the patient's level when with him. They must seek and gain all the outside advice and help they can get but must always remember that the task is one that requires daily, almost hourly attention and therefore is largely their responsibility. Outside help from the doctor, the nurse, or the aphasia therapist can at best be only partial and is usually only advisory.

Today we are only beginning to understand some of the basic problems involved in recovery for the aphasic patient. Each such problem presents a new challenge and requires new hope and new faith to be successfully attacked. What is very sure is that aphasia in most cases needs to be attacked. It will not resolve itself in the great majority of cases. The family must be, in the final analysis, the foundation upon which all recovery must be based.

Chapter 12

DIRECT THERAPY IN RECEPTIVE APHASIA

The preceding chapters have shown the need for an organismic viewpoint toward aphasia. Therapy aimed at total recovery from the effects of the brain injury must also follow the same pathway. Definite consideration must be given to the patient's need to reassume a proper place in life, a place in which he can establish an effective relationship with the society in which he must live and work. While part of this relation can be in terms of insight into his propensities and his limitations, an equal part must be in terms of his language ability. The goals and the medium through which the patient reaches a greater understanding of the world and his place within it are discussed in the many texts on personality and psychotherapy. For the purposes of the present work no one psychotherapeutic school or method is suggested. The therapist must remember, however, that language recovery cannot be expected within a vacuum. The patient must obtain a clear image of self and a rational acceptance of his relationship with the world in which he lives before language recovery can be expected to be maximally successful. Psychological readjustment must be recognized as a necessary part of the therapeutic program in the light of our present knowledge of the behavior characteristics of the brain-injured individual.

With the foregoing recognition, the next chapters deal with the direct language skills that are necessary and some of the techniques that have been found useful in attaining these skills. These methods are proposed with a word of caution. They are not intended as particular steps to be taken with any aphasic patient. Each such individual presents a unique and specific problem that must be considered in the light of his own needs. The techniques and methods discussed in the following pages are, then, only suggestive of a type of approach that has been used with some patients and found successful. From these methods the therapist may be able to construct particular approaches to the individual patient who comes under his care.

For the most part the methods shown will be those used at the beginning of training. The speed with which the steps are taken, the stages of recovery, and the recovery attained differ so widely with the individual that no generalities can be stated. Each patient determines his own speed and the limits of his own recovery. Continuation therapy after the early steps are taken must follow the expressed attitudes of the patient and cannot be developed by the therapist in advance. For example, a patient who shows an alexia may need an initial approach that begins with basic letter-form recognition. From this it may be necessary to go through syllable recognition-span, short word forms, multisyllabic word recognition, and short-phrase, long-phrase and eventually full eye-span word recognition before speed of reading approaches normal. Another patient may well shorten this process after the initial training and go directly from the basic letter recognition to full, short-phrase, or long-phrase eye-span reading. For this reason, no generalities or specific recommendations concerning particular methods will be given. Rather only illustrations of the approaches used and suggestions concerning some of the ways in which they can be used will be offered.

The individual items isolated by the aphasia screening test as shown in Chapter 9 will be dealt with separately. It should be noted that these techniques are rarely used alone but in almost every instance are coupled with others that meet the unique general problem of the patient.

Direct Language Therapy for Agnosia

Agnosia for Visual Form.—The problem here is the failure to recognize simple and common geometrical forms. As expressed in the test, these forms are a square, a cross, and a triangle. Either inability or difficulty in making this recognition may be basic to a failure to recognize letter forms in reading, or it may be isolated and limited to a simple geometrical-form disability. In the former instance the problem is acute and must be dealt with before the fundamental reading problem can be taken up. Where the geometrical form alone is concerned, the problem is frequently not acute and often is not recognized as a disability. In the latter instance therapy is frequently delayed until the need for using form recognition is felt and expressed by the patient. This is most often seen in the later stages of therapy after a considerable degree of recovery has been obtained. When form recognition is found to be basic to the visualization of letters for reading, however, it must be dealt with in the very early stages of training.

Two types of training are suggested for this disability. The first and most generally successful is as follows: The patient is presented with a series of small wooden blocks similar to the geometrical cutouts used on many performance tests. (The Vigotsky or the Healy-Fernald puzzle blocks are useful in this connection.) He is asked to do simple sorting. Thus a series of circles and an equal number of squares of different sizes are presented. As the grouping is achieved, the basic form differences are pointed out. The common name is used for each form and repetition by the patient is requested but not insisted upon. Similar sorting is followed for triangles and crosses. As many two-figure sortings are done as is necessary to show the patient that each physical shape has differentiating characteristics, that size is not a criterion, that only the principle of shape is necessary to make a satisfactory grouping, and that a different name is attached to each group. The grouping process is continued until the patient can at request select the figure named by the therapist from a total grouping of all the many geometrical forms.

It was often found that this procedure was not enough to produce rapid or accurate form discrimination. In those instances where success was difficult, the patient was asked to trace each form or to copy a form presented either on paper or on a blackboard. These attempts were named by the therapist as they were produced by the patient, until by the naming alone the patient could produce the desired form. A third stage of training for the same problem when success was not easily obtained was to have the patient cut out of paper forms drawn by the therapist. In one case it was found to be necessary to have the patient cut the forms out of wood before a basic recognition was obtained. Using only the forms mentioned, it was possible in most cases to obtain a recognition of all geometrical forms. The principle of form recognition followed, no matter what form was presented.

Some patients fail to obtain a sufficient stimulation from the methods described to succeed in the goal of sight recognition of geometrical forms. Since these patients are also unable to visualize the letter forms necessary for reading, it is necessary to devise other means of reducing the problem. A review of the case histories for visual form agnosia of the patients discussed in Chapter 5 showed a common factor among them. The immediate damage to the cortex was either high on the occipital lobe or distal on the parietal lobe of the left hemisphere. Since actual damage to the visual mechanism is found most frequently in these posterior lobe disorders, it was considered that there might be an actual destruction of at least part of the visual pathway. To test this hypothesis, the geometrical forms used were greatly increased in size. Where we had previously been using a maximal two-inch form, each of the figures was increased to approximately twelve inches. The same procedures discussed above were followed, and success was obtained. For this small group of patients, the principle of size added to that of form was necessary for success. From this clue in form recognition a complete language instruction plan can be developed for this type of patient, based upon initial presentation in enlarged size of all the figures necessary.

While a considerable amount of time may be found necessary to overcome this seemingly simple problem, in almost every case the problem can be overcome and no more complex techniques are necessary than the ones described. In the few cases where the form-recognition principle cannot be obtained, there will usually be found a failure to advance in most other visual percepts. A review of the case histories of those patients failing to recognize forms shows that they present a general picture of intellectual impairment. This factor makes therapy of any kind exceedingly difficult.

Visual Number Agnosia.—Patients exhibiting this type of aphasia problem show an inability to recognize numbers presented visually. Thus a fundamental integrative process is affected. Numbers are universally used, are learned early in the child's educational life, and are fundamentally important in any adjustment to life beyond the infantile state. The problem, however, is rarely attacked in the early phases of treatment. During the period of hospital care, when the patient is not ambulatory, the need for a knowledge of numbers is not vital to recovery or to adjustment. As the patient becomes ambulatory, however, the lack of number recognition is commonly felt and is severely debilitating. The usual time for education in the number area is after beginning reading and speech have been accomplished.

Where visual-number recognition is the sole problem, the task can be approached through such devices as writing from dictation, teaching the integers as the letters of an alphabet are taught, by constant reiteration of the spoken number as the digit is copied or traced. It was also found useful to learn the initial digits by rote. In some cases the number of fingers can be used by drawing a facsimile of the patient's hands and assigning a number to each finger. In other cases an interest was developed in a numbered calendar and the digits were learned through the days of the week. It must be remembered that the faculty of number recognition, while basic to a use of numbers, is not identical with use. Often the use of numbers must await recovery of the ability to recognize number form. If it is necessary to teach a sight recognition of the alphabet before reading can be commenced, it is useful to include the teaching of number recognition with that of the alphabet. Where there is a lack of basic form recognition, as in the preceding paragraphs, the learning of the number symbol may be delayed until form recognition is gained. There seems to be a large factor of form recognition in all basic letter and number recognition.

In most of the work a consistent use can be made of the blackboard, with drill and copying of presented number symbols accompanied by verbal naming of each number as it is presented and copied. Many forms of presenting the integers have been used. For some patients a differently colored chalk for each number apparently aids the memory process. Other patients seem to gain their recognition through repetition of the numbers on daily copying in their own workbooks. Still others made a real gain only when numbers were put to some use akin to their interests. Thus one patient who closely identified himself with the sport world learned numbers only when they were used to identify different players on a football and baseball team. Another made the gain through the use of numbers presented on paper money, while still another gained his initial recognition by the identifying numbers on army airplanes. In general, it seems that, for the majority of patients, simple presentation and repetition are sufficient. For those needing additional motivation or stimulation, it may be necessary to seek out interest areas through which the basic learning can be achieved.

Visual Letter Agnosia.—In this area the defect seen is a basic lack of recognition of the letters of the alphabet. In some instances this is seen as the fundamental structure upon which reading is based. In an equal number of instances, however, the problem seems to be limited to the stated recognition of letters of the alphabet, possibly associated with form recognition (see "Visual Form Agnosia" above) and unrelated to meaningful reading. In the former instance the suggestion is made that the difficulty receive immediate attention in the therapeutic process, for reading is one of the most basic language needs of many patients. Where reading is not affected by the disability, it should be treated as part of a form-recognition problem only and brought into therapy only as the need for it arises in the goal searching of the individual patient.

From the foregoing it can be seen that two basic approaches can be used in attacking the problem. Where it is fundamental to reading, the meaningfulness of the letter form should be stressed. The letter form is taught as part of a unit which produces a meaningful word. It is usually found that patients can learn the alphabet by rote without progressing toward the goal of reading. The goal in these patients is that of reading for meaning, and attempts to teach the alphabet by rote, expecting a transfer to meaningfulness, have been found to be laborious and in most instances have proved to be quite futile.

As direct steps in training, the following procedures have been found to be useful. Using picture forms cut out of papers and magazines which illustrate initial letters, the patient is taught a series of words, such as *A* for "animal," *B* for "baby," etc. The letters are copied from a visual presentation, either on a blackboard or on paper. Where necessary they are first traced by the patient. As the letter is copied or traced, the picture illustrating the object whose whole name began with the letter is presented and the name is spoken and written by the instructor. A complete alphabet can be developed following this procedure. For the most part, aphasic patients need only a start in order to go through the entire alphabet. Most patients who are shown the first five or six letters in this form are able to build their own alphabets with only a minimum of difficulty. When consistent errors are seen in alphabet reproduction, they should be corrected by the instructor. Through simple experimentation it may be found that color will add to the ease of learning, and all pictures then are presented in color. It may also be found that there is more rapid learning when pictures can be selected that motivate the patients by their content. For one patient it was noted that a paste-in workbook kept by him in which he posted his own illustrative pictures was a helpful motivating device. For another patient, Hilaire Belloc's *A Moral Alphabet*[1] was found to be useful. This type of book has a rather high difficulty level and often is found to be too complex for most patients.

One of the most difficult of all the problems of direct language training is well illustrated in this area. It is given here in some detail because it applies as well to almost every other phase of the therapeutic process. Most aphasic patients are adults. They are capable of, and in most instances do, think and act on an adult level. The type of difficulty they have, however, requires work-material on

---

[1] H. Belloc, *A Moral Alphabet* (London: Gerald Duckworth & Co., Ltd., 1932).

the most fundamental level. Almost no printed material exists that combines mature thought with fundamental form. For this reason almost the entire material load must be constructed by the therapist or by the patient. Usually this problem falls to the former. A workbook illustrating simple fundamentals in material that might be interesting to the adult is badly needed. One student working on the problem has been over three years trying to develop such a workbook with only minimal success. The author has found it necessary to help his patients develop such material separately on almost every occasion. This presents many problems, but the actual discovery of the material by the patient and the construction of the workbooks has been found to be a helpful instructional aid in itself. Most patients take considerable pride in their ability to find and learn material that has not previously been used. This seems extremely helpful in maintaining individual motivation. It is, however, extremely slow and time-consuming. Most of the workbooks developed by patients are found to be incomplete and carried out only as far as that patient needs to go in learning the particular task before him.

In general, it should be stated that the larger goal of reading should constantly be kept in mind when working with the patient whose letter-form recognition problem is thought to be basic to reading. This may serve in part to delay recovery of letter-form recognition but usually will be found to speed the beginning of reading. Where the problem is a part of the form-recognition function, letter recognition can best be taught through techniques similar to those described above. In this area the recognition is gained most easily through such methods as sorting cutout letters, copying forms on the board or on paper, selecting a particular letter and crossing it out in large printed material, and playing such letter games as "Bingo" or "Lotto" with a printed form which presents to the patient a multiple-letter choice.

This latter game was developed for a number of patients who seemed to learn most things best in competition with others, although it has also been used with single patients with some success. The therapist takes a sheet of ordinary typewriter paper and rules it off so that a number of equal-sized squares appear. Depending upon the difficulty desired, these squares can be as many as twenty to the page or as few as nine. In each square a different letter is printed. (Where form recognition as well as letter recognition is being trained, the squares can contain the geometrical forms such as circle, square, etc.) The instructor then writes a letter on the board, or calls it, and the patient attempts to find that letter on his paper. The first patient to complete a row is declared winner. An extension of this procedure was found to be useful for number recognition. As will be seen later, it can also be adapted to many other areas of the language act. Variations of this method, using words, pictures, and other stimulating symbols were tried in the other areas with some success.

It should be noted that there is a marked difference between rote learning and repetition of the alphabet and letter-form recognition. Many patients who are almost global in their disability retain serial speech. They can count with ease if once started and can also repeat most of the alphabet. Actual form recognition of the letters of the alphabet can only be said to be learned and possessed by the patient when he can recognize letters given at random.

Visual Word Agnosia (Alexia).—The inability or disability shown by most aphasic patients in comprehension of the printed word is probably the best known and most widely discussed of all the language handicaps. Too frequently the term "alexia" is misused in this connection. For the present purpose it is intended that it be used in its textbook meaning only, that is, the reading disability due directly to injury to the cerebral cortex. In the extensive educational literature dealing with reading and with remedial reading, the term has come to mean almost any disorder of reading. Because of the importance of reading in the educative process for all children, the subject has been studied from many viewpoints. The aim of the present section will be to present some of the initial steps that can be taken in assisting brain-injured patients, especially those who show a complete or very severe reading problem, and in addition some of the principles of reading instruction and a fairly wide bibliography on the problem for related reading.

It should be pointed out that, in most work with aphasic adults, the therapist is largely concerned with the beginning process. When a residual remains, it may be found most satisfactory to turn to a trained remedial reading tutor for assistance in reducing the later stages of difficulty.

Where the problem is a complete one, it is usually necessary to begin with the suggestions offered earlier under "Visual Form Agnosia" and "Visual Letter Agnosia." Both of these areas may be fundamental to the reading problem seen. When the patient is able to recognize forms and letters, the task remains of training the ability to gain sight recognition of whole words and phrases so that comprehension and retention can be obtained.

Dolch [2] lists five major steps in remedial reading:

1. Go back where he is.
2. Build sight vocabulary and speed recognition.
3. Teach self-help sounding.
4. Develop comprehension.
5. Secure much interesting reading at present level.

These five points are basic to any approach to the alexic patient. It is axiomatic to say that the therapist should determine the patient's reading level through examination and begin training at that point. The sight vocabulary as a basic step can be checked, as Dolch indicates, against such standard forms as Gray's *Oral Reading Paragraphs* [3] or the basic sight vocabulary test. [4] These tests will show the retained reading vocabulary upon which the patient's more advanced reading must grow. Even though a number of words are retained in a sight vocabulary, there must be speed of recognition for retention and comprehension. It may be wise to drill for speed of presently retained words before extending the basic sight vocabulary. Instant recognition is necessary for advancement of the reading skill.

Sounding of words as advised in step 3 above can be taught through any form of phonetics. Some writers advise teaching the sounds as they occur in simple words, starting always with the first consonant and proceeding through the short vowels to medial and final sounds. The author has experienced little difficulty in sounding instruction with aphasic patients if they can recall the phonetic alphabet. Many patients, however, are unable to sound out or spell words, while they can gain whole-word recognitions. Where this is true, omit individual sound training and stay on the word level. Several patients with visual word difficulty have learned to read easily and rapidly without being able to master the individual letters or sounds of their native language. Whenever the patient shows extreme difficulty or withdrawal from the sound level, the short-single-syllable-word level with meaning attached should be tried as the initial stage of training after basic sight recognition.

In working toward comprehension, the patient should repeat the meaning of short phrases immediately after reading them. It is

---

[2] E. W. Dolch, *A Manual for Remedial Reading* (Champaign, Ill.: The Garrard Press, 1945).

[3] William S. Gray, *Oral Reading Paragraphs* (Bloomington, Ill.: Public School Publishing Co.).

[4] E. W. Dolch, *Basic Sight Word Test* (Champaign, Ill.: The Garrard Press).

best not to start with delayed recall, as this is an extremely difficult task for the alexic patient. A workbook of selected material for each patient, based upon his interest and comprehension level, should be developed and added to. There are no all-useful books or work material available for adults that have come to the author's attention. Parrot-like repetition should be avoided. Sometimes the paragraph rather than the sentence is the best level for training. The therapist should not insist on accuracy, but stress and encourage any effort to express meaning levels from read material. While retelling is of great importance, it is frequently an impossible level for the aphasic patient, since verbal areas are often affected. Any form of retelling may be used, whether it be by words, actions, writing, or simple gesture. While the ability to select the most important things in a given reading selection is an important function in the reading process, it must be remembered that aphasic patients frequently are unable to abstract. This leads to extreme problems in retention and comprehension of what is expected from most readers. Any meaning that is even remotely connected with the material should be accepted.

Finally, the admonition of Dolch mentioned above to secure much material at the patient's present level may be one of the most difficult tasks faced by the therapist. Material that is of interest, that will motivate and stimulate the patient and still be on his level, will often tax the ingenuity of the best therapists. The therapist should not miss an opportunity to add to his collection of material. Current magazines, adult texts rewritten for children, and therapist-rewritten familiar stories are the best sources.

A number of books other than those previously cited have been found helpful by the author in formulating the methodology used.[5] The books cited are not only directly valuable for their content but also for their own bibliographies. Where extreme difficulty is found in obtaining improvement, the author has invariably turned to the specialist in remedial reading for assistance. In this area at least there has been sufficient research and experimentation so that assistance is not too difficult to obtain. Many aphasic patients, however, do not need special reading tutors or instructors. As their other problems in language are met, it is frequently found that the type of instruction discussed above is sufficient to get the patient started on

---

[5] Grace Fernald, *Remedial Reading Techniques* (New York: McGraw-Hill Book Co., Inc., 1943). Arthur Gates, *Improvement in Reading* (New York: The Macmillan Co., 1947), p. 108. William S. Gray, *On Their Own in Reading* (Chicago: Scott, Foresman & Co., 1948).

the road to reading recovery. Practice and use are of greatest assistance in the complete resolution of the problem.

Visual Size Agnosia.—This is one of the less frequently observed receptive problems. While almost never seen in isolation, it sometimes is associated with the visual form agnosia discussed above and may play a definite part in reading difficulties. The inability to differentiate different-sized symbols or objects may lead to considerable practical embarrassment in manual vocations. For working tasks which require the use of tools of differing sizes, or as in one case studied by the author of a printer who needed to select different sizes of type, the inability to select the proper size led to immediate unemployment. The problem presents a special cue to certain reading disabilities. Most reading material is presented in print of a few sizes, and even in children's books rarely goes beyond this limited range. The patient with a visual size agnosia is frequently unable to differentiate letters which look alike unless the size is magnified beyond the limits of his disability. One patient who at first was thought to have an alexia was found to possess normal reading ability when the print size was increased to five inches. Whenever the element of size agnosia is present, it is necessary to plan the entire visual training program with special material designed to offset the problem, otherwise therapy is doomed to failure even though the patient be re-educable.

Direct methods of approach to the problem as used by the author are two in number. For the patient mentioned above whose alexia seemed based upon the size component, it was found to be of value to decrease the size of the material presented by successively small decrements. Thus after the patient demonstrated that he could read satisfactorily with the material presented at a normal distance from the eye (fixation point twelve inches) and each letter raised to five-inch size, he was tried with slightly smaller letters. The first reduction attempted was one-half inch, but the letters were found to be too small unless the material was brought close to the eyes, when it blurred so that only imperfect attempts were attained. The material size was then increased to four and three-fourths inches, and after some effort the patient was able to succeed with fair speed. The next reduction made was one-fourth inch, and the patient again succeeded after some ten days of trial and effort. The next reduction was one-eighth inch, and success with normal speed and accuracy was obtained in a period of seven days. Following that attempt, each succeeding week found the patient able to reduce the size necessary for easy reading by one-eighth inch. At the time of discharge, fourteen months after the beginning of therapy, the patient was reading regular-sized print.

The above description does not adequately cover the total problem, for as reading was presented in larger print and success was obtained, so too was it necessary for the patient to write with larger-sized print and script or the writing was found to be unintelligible. Writing, therefore, followed the same process of reduction in size as did reading. Occasionally one would lag behind the other. When this did occur, it was found to be most helpful to retard the progression until both were at an equal level. This seemed to help the patient maintain interest, understand his progress, and gauge his improvement.

The same technique was tried on three other patients and seemed to be beneficial to each. One patient who was in the process of recovery at the time the Aphasia Center discussed in Chapter 5 was closed continued on his own at home. A letter received from him approximately nine months after leaving the direct training program showed a complete return to regular reading and writing. The letter itself was probably the best evidence, since it was in regular-sized script without guiding or size lines.

One patient, however, did not respond to the treatment outlined, and it was necessary to devise another approach to the problem for him. While reading was affected by the problem, it was impossible to stimulate this patient with written material. A hand-worker and almost a nonreader prior to his injury, he found himself unable to concentrate on any of the material presented. However, an excellent rapport had been established between the patient and the occupational therapist. His visual agnosia displayed itself in the shop at every turn. When he attempted to work with plastics, his material would always be cut to the wrong size. The top of one box that he made was three-quarters of an inch larger than the box itself. His attempted selection of tools always left him puzzled. One size of file was used for a particular operation, but he would invariably bring or select either a size too large or a size too small. Therapy for this patient was developed by using objects and blocks of differing sizes.

As was indicated above for the other patients, the technique used was the simple one of decreasing size by successive decrements. Using blocks first, a series was presented where the differential was as great as two inches. Thus a set of two sizes of blocks was presented, six being three-inch cubes and six one-inch cubes. The patient was asked to sort them into two equal piles. When a two-inch differential was used, the patient succeeded at the third trial. After success had been obtained a series of times with ease and speed, the larger blocks were reduced to two-and-one-half-inch cubes. With this differential the patient succeeded in making a successful sorting only once in twenty trials. Each day as a part of his training program the blocks were presented and the patient would attempt his sorting. Since success was so difficult to obtain, the differential was increased to one and three-quarter inches, that is the larger blocks were made two and three-quarter inch cubes. This brought about an increase in accuracy. After two weeks of daily trials, the patient was able to succeed on each trial. Following this the decrement used was one-fourth inch, and the sizes were changed as soon as the patient indicated his ability by successful sorting. After the patient could differentiate cubes differing by one-fourth inch, he was tried with lines and squares presented on the blackboard. It was found that the differential again had to be increased, not to the two-inch difference, but to at least one inch. Again by successive decrements the patient succeeded in differentiating lines and squares and later circles and other geometrical figures that differed in size by as little as one-eighth inch. From the figure differentials the patient found it an easy step to differentiate letters of a typical reading size and went on to a greater success in reading. It was also noted that with little practice after this the patient could differentiate other objects in the shop, although their sizes were much alike.

The author wishes to stress the importance of the size agnosias and the fundamental and debilitating nature of the problem when it is present. At the same time it is not proposed that the methods outlined above are in any sense the only approaches to the problem. They are the only two methods tried by the author with any degree of success.

Visual Color Agnosia.—The inability of certain aphasic adults to recognize colors has been mentioned many times in the literature. Kleist, Gelb and Goldstein, Potzl, and others have commented upon the brain-injured patient's color recognition difficulty.[6] It is differentiated from color blindness in that in the latter there is a tendency to miscall or fail to recognize the difference between colors. In the aphasic patient there is no miscalling of colors, no reversal of the

---

[6] T. Weisenburg and K. McBride, *Aphasia* (New York: The Commonwealth Fund, Division of Publications, 1935).

red-green color combinations, no all-blue perceptions as reported in descriptions of the color-blind. The aphasic patient seems unable to recognize that color is a part of the percept. His Gestalt is incomplete in the color sense. Actually, this would seem to be a real blindness for color. While the diagnosticians have been free to indicate the presence of the difficulty, none of the sparse literature on therapy mentions retraining in this area.

While no patients in the author's experience have been completely lacking in color discrimination, those that have shown a disability in this particular have responded to fairly simple teaching techniques. By using common objects and foods of many colors, it is usually not difficult by conditioning procedures to teach a basic recognition of color. Thus, as other words are regained, through verbal techniques which will be described later, the colors of common objects are added as additional clues toward simple recognition. Thus, an orange is presented as a fruit, as being round, as being edible, and as being orange in color. A tomato is differentiated from an orange by name and by color, with the other properties more or less in common. A grapefruit has a different size, a different name, a different taste, and a different color. A banana differs in size from an orange in shape, in taste, and in color. A green grape, a blue grape, a black walnut, a green pear, etc., are all useful to show the differing properties, one of which is color. By ascribing the proper color originally and reviewing the names with these properties, recognition can often be obtained on each of the named categories, and color is always included. After the patient can differentiate the common fruits by color, the exercises are extended to other nonedible objects like chalk for white, black for the color of the blackboard, brown for the desk, green in the drapes, etc. Through this learning process all but one of the author's patients succeeded in recovering his color-recognition sense. This one patient failed to achieve a resolution of his difficulty, although many other approaches were made.

When the color sense is lacking, one of the most stimulating of simple teaching methods is lost. Many patients learned their first words for verbal expression and achieved their first word recognitions in reading through the medium of the colored picture. Here color can be used positively as a stimulating device. Where visual color agnosia is present, these methods are futile and it is only with the resolution of the disability that colored pictures can be used. It is believed that this tends to keep the recovery pattern of some of the patients below the expected speed of recovery.

Audio-visuo-kinetic Agnosia.—As the name implies, this problem is more complex than the previously described visual agnosias. In the sphere here described is man's ability to recognize actions seen or heard by means of the movement that accompanies the action. In the test form, the act of pursing the lips for whistling should be recognized as that act as distinguished from any other act, just as the act of raising the hand to indicate the command "halt" or the gesture of the hand that accompanies the request to move forward. When the perceived sign, either auditory as in whistling or visual as in the case of a traffic policeman's gesture, does not convey meaning to the individual, he is said to have an audio-visuo-kinetic agnosia. The actions described can be seen to be consistently embarrassing and very debilitating to the patient.

Therapeusis should follow very direct conditioning methods. The patient needs to be given many examples of each of the combined acts and asked to relate the meaning attached. It was found that the symbols attached to the many common gestures could be learned by the majority of patients in a comparatively short time by observing repeated demonstrations either by the instructor or by other patients. Repetition, practice, and experience served in almost every case to obviate the problem. Where it did not, an increased number of examples was used, even such simple ones as the raised hand to indicate a desire to write on the blackboard or to recite, or to call the attention of the instructor to the patient's lesson. The number of small examples that could be used in everyday life was found to be sufficient to give the practice necessary. In some cases it was found to be of value to teach the manual code used universally in automobile driving, while for other patients it was necessary to add the printed word indicating the desired action whenever the problems were posed.

While this problem seems to have been largely overlooked in the literature of therapy, it proved to be of so stimulating character and so closely related to life for most patients that it was frequently used with patients even when the problem itself as a separate agnosia did not seem to exist.

Auditory Verbal Agnosia.—The major receptive disability of the aphasic adult is in comprehension of the spoken word. In terms of differential diagnosis it is important to recognize the aphasic disturbance as apart from (a) deafness and (b) general intellectual impairment. When these two complicating factors have been ruled out by test and observation, the degree of loss of comprehension remains as the cortical disability of integrating aural stimuli. Originally this disorder was defined by Wernicke [7] as "true" aphasia, and it has been the subject of a long and extensive body of research defining its limits. At one time called "word-deafness," one form of the disorder was described by Froeschels as being present when "inner speech was fully intact . . . only comprehension of speech is entirely destroyed." [8] In this form it is necessary to retrain understanding only. The more commonly seen auditory verbal agnosia, however, as described by Wernicke [9] is characterized by defective comprehension of speech with disturbances in voluntary speech, but with a retained ability to imitate words. It has been the author's experience that patients showing this problem have all gradations between comparatively normal speech production and a total lack of that facility, between a total lack of comprehension and a partial lack of the ability to understand spoken words, and between a retained ability to imitate and an apparent total lack of imitative ability.

One factor which stands out in all these patients is their almost total lack of self-criticism of speech. Whatever speech they attempt seems to satisfy them. This appears to indicate that consciousness of the speech act is entirely gained from the speech produced, rather than from any internal or cortical conscious awareness of speech while it is being spoken. The patient's inability to correct his own speech places an especially heavy burden on the therapist, for not only must comprehension be regained but failure and success at production must be externally shown.

In this area of disturbance more than any other must the total available resources of the patient be utilized. Where auditory stimuli are meaningless, the patient must be approached from the tactile-auditory, the visual-auditory, the kinetic-auditory, and the combined visuo-tactile-kinetic-auditory. It should be noted that in each of the proposed approaches the auditory function is an integrated part of the training. The end product is not an ability to develop a substitute for hearing, nor by circuitous methods to hope for a transfer of training, but to redevelop in the patient his use of the disturbed auditory function.

As mentioned earlier in the section on alexia, the aphasia therapist can call upon existing techniques used for other nonaphasic disorders. The body of instructional material developed for training the deaf patient will be of considerable value in some cases. Lip

---

[7] Weisenburg and McBride, op. cit., p. 10.
[8] E. Froeschels, *Speech Therapy* (Boston: Expression Co., 1933), p. 123.
[9] Weisenburg and McBride, op. cit., p. 10.

reading or phonetic instruction in which the patient learns to follow the observable movements of the articulatory musculature may be of great assistance. Any good text in speech pathology will indicate the methods of articulatory instruction. The author recommends for this purpose, West, Kennedy, and Carr's *Rehabilitation of Speech*,[10] Van Riper's *Speech Correction*,[11] and Berry and Eisenson's *The Defective in Speech*.[12] There are also several good texts on lip reading, such as Goldstein's *The Acoustic Method*[13] and others. Fernald's *Remedial Reading Techniques*[14] is replete with suggestions on the kinesthetic approach to speech and other language functions. For direct language instruction the techniques advised also follow the tactile approach, in which the patient is asked to touch the therapist's laryngeal musculature as well as the facial structure during speech and thus gain a direct contactual picture of the speech act. This will assist in showing the patient the difference between the voiced and unvoiced sounds when the larynx is palpated during speech, between nasal and oral sounds when the nose and cheeks are palpated, and between plosives and continuants when the oral structures are contacted. One very general comment for the therapist is that success will be obtained only when the material used is at the interest level of the patient. Motivation and stimulation are almost impossible unless the patient has been studied carefully from this viewpoint.

One patient who lacked understanding to a high degree had been a housewife for over twenty-five years. Her interests centered in the making of a home. Purely academic material failed to maintain her interest beyond the presenting period. When, however, instruction was attempted, with the names for the ingredients of a cake, she was interested, tried much harder, did not lapse into her consistent futility pattern, and succeeded in obtaining a beginning understanding of the use of language.

To make this point doubly clear, since it is so important, note the approach used with another patient. This patient, a woman of approximately the same age as the preceding one, had had a pretraumatic life on a high professional education level. She could obtain comprehension only through the use of such material as events

---

[10] Robert West, *et al., Rehabilitation of Speech* (rev. ed.; New York: Harper & Bros., 1947).

[11] C. Van Riper, *Speech Correction* (New York: Prentice-Hall, Inc., 1947).

[12] M. Berry and J. Eisenson, *The Defective in Speech* (New York: Appleton-Century-Crofts, Inc., 1947).

[13] Max Goldstein, *The Acoustic Method* (St. Louis: Laryngoscope Press, 1939).

[14] *Op. cit.*

in history, explanation surrounding current events as pictured in magazines and newspapers, and the like.

The therapist must be alert to all forms of stimulating material. Attention and concentration defects, the simplest common denominators of brain-injured adults, will present an exceedingly difficult barrier to success unless they are considered constantly when the type of material to be used is selected. While this is true in every form of education and re-education, it seems to have special importance with patients showing auditory verbal agnosias because of the extreme difficulty of direct communication with these patients.

By using every possible combination of stimuli for the defective auditory sense, it is possible to obviate a considerable part of even the most serious auditory verbal defects. For emphasis a few of the direct approaches used are listed here. One patient was given a series of pictures and was asked to write the word name that symbolized each illustration. (The Dolch picture cards [15] are of considerable value in this approach.) When it was found that the spoken name for the picture was meaningless, the patient was asked to copy the printed title. As the word was completed, the name was repeated, and the patient was asked to repeat it. Later the picture alone was presented as the word was reiterated by the therapist. After a series of pictures and words was presented, the patient was found to have learned that the spoken word coincided with the printed word. With closure of this Gestalt obtained, the patient without more than simple review was able to produce the word from a simple showing of the picture and the reiteration of the word name. Following considerable success at this level, the word name alone was repeated and the patient selected the correct picture from a series. This was accompanied by a repetition by the patient of the correct word as the picture was selected. Using nouns only at the onset, verbs were added after success had been obtained on the nominative level. Adjectives and adverbs followed in order with rapid success. Sentences followed phrases, and eventually slow and clearly enunciated speech became the only necessary stimulus.

Another patient could only obtain meaning at the initial stages if she could handle the object named and if for her it had some old familiar usage. Thus, the names of tableware, like "fork," "spoon," and "knife," were the beginning words in her comprehension vocabulary. It has become increasingly evident to the author, as more and more of the progress of these patients is reviewed, that methodology can be described only in terms of the individual patient. While the

---

[15] E. W. Dolch, *A Manual for Remedial Reading.*

methods used may be easily categorized as serving a particular function or as retraining a particular language facet, what the therapist must do is to apply the material that is closest to the life-pattern of the patient if continued progress and success are to be obtained.

Auditory verbal agnosia, despite the apparent simplicity of the above-described techniques, is without question one of the most difficult of all the aphasic disturbances to correct. Time appears to be a matter of little consideration in the process. It may take from one to several months to obtain insight and closure in any of the steps or stages of development described above. What has appeared consistently, however, is the fact that these patients seem to learn by stages rather than by slight, successive steps. Absolute failure at any one level for a period of months may be followed by a very rapid accretion of comprehended language after the first few Gestalts are obtained. It is important to stress this factor, for in no other area of aphasia re-education is the need for perseverance on the part of the therapist so necessary. Failure of a particular approach should be no reason for abandoning it. If the therapist believes that the proper avenue is being explored and if the patient continues to evidence interest and effort even though complaining of an inability to succeed, the therapy should continue. When the analysis leads the therapist to believe that the avenue is the correct one, an approach should be abandoned only if the patient cannot be stimulated to continue. Keep changing the stimulating material, use different picture forms or different objects, shift from tactual to kinetic to visual stimuli, but keep returning to the simple and obvious examples within the framework of the patient's interest.

Auditory Music Agnosia (Amusia).—Froeschels defines receptive musical agnosia as "inability to perceive certain musical elements or complexes . . . he may be unable to recognize music, to remember it, to know what instruments are being played, what kind of emotions are being expressed, whether the tempo is fast or slow, what rhythm is used, whether the reproduction is correct or not . . . the disorders described usually appear combined in various ways." [16] This disability is often a source of considerable concern to the patient whose previous vocation or avocation was concerned with music in any serious form. For the average patient, however, music was found to be a bypath of the pretraumatic life, a means of enjoyment rather than a serious study. For these patients, the presence of a receptive amusia was rarely a matter of concern, certainly not rank-

---

[16] E. Froeschels, *op. cit.,* p. 94.

ing in any sense with the speaking, reading, or writing problems that occurred concurrently with the musical disability. Most often, when the problem was discovered by examination, it had not occurred to the patient as a problem. Following the general approach to the aphasic adult of treating what the patient considered most important in his constellation of difficulties, the musical disability was very often not approached in the early days of therapy but left to the later periods, when more refined disorders became a matter of concern.

In well over a hundred cases of severe aphasia seen in adults, the author has never seen a serious case of musical disability in a patient where the comprehension of music was important. For suggestions in therapy we therefore again turn to Froeschels' work. This author relates the techniques to be used in the following way.

The therapy of musical disorders must be adapted to the needs of the individual case and consists in a kind of remedial retraining in music. An exact examination is absolutely necessary in order to find the basic difficulties which impair the patient's performance. In any case we should go back to his primary impairments and try to remove them by retraining the basic capacities which have been affected. This treatment must be carried out on lines similar to those used in the treatment of aphasics. A thorough musical education on the part of the therapist is an absolute necessity. If he is not an accomplished pianist, he should seek the collaboration of such a musician . . . the greatest care is to be taken not to exhaust the patient or to depress him by making him feel his own deficiencies.[17]

Goldstein makes the distinction between singing and speaking very pointedly. He believes that

. . . singing is likely to remain in spite of speech disturbances when it is an activity closely connected with the patient's affective life. Under such conditions, the song is not representative speech, but a "series speech" performance expressive of feeling, like a prayer.[18]

In many of the aphasias studied by the present writer where there appeared to be marked inability to recognize music and an equally marked inability to speak, there was this retained ability to sing simple compositions that were apparently stereotypes from the pretraumatic state of the patient. With Goldstein, the author believes that they are not representative speech. Every attempt to use these retained words from musical compositions for voluntary speech were unsuccessful.

---

[17] *Ibid.,* p. 96 ff.
[18] K. Goldstein, "Die Lokalization in der Grosshirnrinde," *Handbuch. der normalen und pathologischen Physiologie,* X (1927), 796.

Music was widely used in setting the background tone of the general therapeutic situation for inpatients in the Aphasic Center discussed earlier. After a consistent exposure to music of different types for a period of several months, it was found that even those patients who had been found to have receptive amusic defects were able to select the kind of music they preferred for relaxation. Since the direct use of music of any kind was not found satisfactory for teaching the other language problems, however, music played only a subordinate background role in the general therapeutic situation.

Auditory Number Agnosia.—In common with other auditory defects of comprehension, a number of patients have been seen who have a distinct problem in being unable to comprehend spoken numbers. This disorder was seen in many instances where other receptive defects were not evidenced. The over-all number-comprehension problem is found in many aphasic adults, and the ability to hear a numerical statement and yet be unable to recognize the numbers involved is a very common one. The use of numbers and simple calculations that affect the patient's everyday living are so common that the inability to use them is a severe handicap to these patients. The simple making of change, the ordinary budgetary problems of making a restricted income last over a period of time, the location of hospital wards by number, the use of the telephone where numbers must be dialed, and a myriad other instances can be related where the problem may affect the everyday living of the aphasic adult. Despite this, the author has found that approaching the auditory number agnosias in the early stages of training has proved most unsatisfactory. The complexities of learning in this area are evidently too severe and the integrations necessary too complex to permit an early training process. For this reason, teaching numbers has usually been delayed until there is some return of language in other spheres. In the general problem of teaching numbers, the retention and use of numbers heard rather than seen are found to be the most difficult. Consequently auditory training on numbers and their use has usually followed visual number training or has been taught simultaneously.

A distinct difference is seen between the actual retention of counting serially and the use of numbers. Many patients as described originally by Jackson[19] can count the digits with great ease just as they have been seen to be able to recall whole musical composi-

---

[19] J. H. Jackson, "Reprint of Some of J. Hughlings Jackson's Papers on Affection of Speech," *Brain*, XXXVIII (1915), 36–39.

tions, but they are frequently unable to use these numbers purposively. In fact the use of numbers has been found to have almost no relation to counting ability, and arithmetical ability cannot be recovered through building on a retained number series.

Therapeutically, training can begin with simple auditory number recognition through the simple objects familiar to the patient, such as the number of fingers on each hand, the addition of the two hands, the subtraction of one hand from two, the number of objects on a desk top, etc. From these simple beginnings it is found to be of value to follow some of the procedures advised in remedial arithmetic books. The author has found Fernald's *Remedial Techniques in Basic School Subjects* [20] to be most useful in suggesting methods and approaches that appeal to some patients. In every instance of training, the visual and auditory senses have been combined, even though one of the abilities is retained. Again, the caution seems necessary that we do not depend upon transfer of training from the visual to the auditory. The patient who can use numbers that are presented visually will not develop from this ability an auditory number sense. There must be a real combination of the visual and the auditory and the progression of difficulty must be based upon success obtained in both areas.

Goldstein [21] pointed out that a good deal of the patient's problem in calculation may be due to his inability to recognize the symbols necessary for carrying out simple arithmetical tasks. The same type of problem has been observed in the auditory area, where patients are unable to use the spoken symbol for computation. Thus, the words "plus," "minus," "divided by," and "multiplied by" do not convey meaning on an auditory verbal agnosia level with special reference to numerical usage.

Re-education in this area should follow the suggestions given earlier. The auditory pattern should be combined with a visual presentation. Where that is unsuccessful, the patient should move objects tactually to coincide with the spoken command. The absolute symbol should be taught first; a later stage of training can be the recognition of the number in practical problems. For the day-by-day usage of numbers where computation may or may not enter in, it will be found most useful to illustrate the problem with practical tasks given either in written or oral form. For one patient whose pretraumatic life included the running of a grocery store, it

---

[20] *Op. cit.*, pp. 213–55.
[21] Kurt Goldstein, *Aftereffects of Brain Injuries in War* (New York: Grune & Stratton, Inc., 1942), p. 206.

was necessary to set up a practice situation in which he actually handled at request a series of objects, like the number of bananas that made up a pound, the number of packages of cigarettes in a carton, etc. By continued use the patient was able to recover his sense of listening to numbers and using them easily and purposively. It is of interest that this same device proved to be so lacking in motivating force to other patients that it was abandoned after the original patient had achieved his goal. To provide life situations for other patients, however, it was found to be of value to have them simulate purchases in the first patient's store, requesting a particular number of objects or responding to the storekeeper when he asked them for the number of a particular object that they wanted.

For a number of patients in the inpatient situation described earlier, the auditory number agnosia was resolved through card-playing. It was found that the patients could most easily be stimulated through such card games as poker and rummy. While the particular inpatient situation, the army hospital, banned poker-playing for money, it was permitted as a therapeutic device. Some eight or ten patients played a nightly game of poker, and though they began at a stage in their recovery when almost no speech was available to them, they managed through sign or gesture to indicate the number of cards they wanted in the particular form of the game called draw poker. The patient suffering from a form of number agnosia was observed to request often a number of cards other than the number actually desired. On correction by the other patients, he would learn that if he wished to discard three cards, he needed to request an equal number to make up the total of five. Since the dealer also might suffer from an auditory number agnosia, it required a considerable degree of watchfulness on the player's part to indicate that the wrong number of cards was being dealt.

In still another way these card games assisted in producing the interests and pressures necessary for learning. While originally the men played for fun, that is without money, this soon became boring and the stimulus of playing for money was added. This addition proved most therapeutic, for every error that affected other players was checked by those other players and every error that affected the immediate player cost him money. Through this most elemental money sense it was found that numbers were learned at a rate that far outstripped other forms of learning language. While no rules were established by the therapist, it was an unwritten law that gestures would be used only when words could not be expressed. The men took to this form of training avidly and continued to display a considerable interest in it throughout their hospitalization and training program.

Another adult patient was found to learn the auditory sense of numbers by playing a simple two-handed card game called "rummy." By calling out each card as it was played, by requesting cards from the discard pile by number, by denominating the sequences of cards as they were played, the patient learned to use numbers *he heard* with comparative ease. Other patients found it necessary to return to such learning behavior as the beginning multiplication tables before they could progress in their number sense, while still others were able to master numbers in the use stage without ever being able to succeed in the rote use of the tables. Again, it must be stressed how individual the approach must be in working with any phase of the aphasic disorder.

Tactile Agnosia.—Defined by Weisenburg as " . . . difficulty in the recognition of objects or forms by touch," [22] the tactile problems seen in aphasic adults rarely impede progress toward language recovery. Since touch alone is rarely used as a teaching method but is almost always accompanied by either visual or auditory stimuli, the patient with tactile agnosia depends upon his other senses for his instructional cues. Where the problem is most debilitating is in the patient whose visual and auditory avenues are affected. For these adults, the tactile pathway needs to be used very extensively. Where there is also a tactile defect, this additional block considerably hinders recovery. Total therapy as proposed in these pages depends to some degree upon the use of as many clues to learning as possible, and the tactile one is frequently called upon to aid in presenting the best possible imagery to the patient. Before the therapist begins to call upon the ability to learn or to retain images through contact with familiar object forms as suggested in earlier paragraphs, the extent of disability in this area must be evaluated and given due consideration.

Direct therapy for disturbances of function in the tactile area is rarely given. In only one of the author's patients was this particular avenue explored with any degree of consistent effort. This patient suffered a head injury to the left temporal and occipital regions. He showed a marked loss in retaining visual and auditory stimuli. Upon examination it was found that the best retained receptive area was the tactual function, although serious delimitation was seen in that area as well. Since no instruction was possible through the

---

[22] Weisenburg and McBride, *op. cit.,* p. 106.

usual media of eye and ear, the patient was drilled on form recognition by daily contacts with common objects. Thus, a coin was placed in his hand, and he was asked to name it, to draw it, to insert it in the correct opening of a structure with many similar-sized openings. (A coin box similar to that used by streetcar conductors was used here.) After he was able to select the proper-sized opening and the verbal symbol for the particular coin had been learned through reiteration and response repetition, he was asked to select different coins by touch until he could differentiate the coins by a combination of the spoken request plus his sense of touch and feeling. This led to an extension of the exercise to other objects such as pencils, rulers, etc. Differences were explained in terms of size, length, thickness, and weight. Each new object was presented both by name and by tactual contact. Through a continuation of this process, a beginning touch and auditory plus visual vocabulary was started. Through conditioning the patient was in time able to recognize the object without touching it, and further instruction was given visually and aurally. A modified form of this procedure was used in a number of cases. Sufficient success was obtained so that other methods in this area were not necessary.

Body Agnosia (Topagnosia or Autotopagnosia).—Pick first described this condition as a ". . . loss of the body schema." [23] It is most commonly displayed in patients showing a generalized receptive disorder and is considered as a part of the disorder called *asteriagnosia* or the inability to gain recognizable impressions from the surface of the body. It also has a close resemblance to the specialized agnosia of Gerstmann called *Fingeragnosia* or the inability to name or indicate given fingers at command. Loss of body schema is seen when the patient is unable to differentiate his right from his left side or to recognize objects or forms in their spatial relationship to his own body. In our civilization where directions are given so frequently in terms of right and left, where an individual needs to place so many objects in their proper relationship to himself, especially in urban living, the presence of a body agnosia can be extremely debilitating.

Training procedures for the patient with this defect need to be practical in the extreme. Actual drill of left and right or estimates of relationship spatially will be found to be quite futile. Success has been achieved in the author's experience only when the patient was continuously placed in situations of either actual or simulated im-

---

[23] *Ibid.,* p. 108.

portance. Recognizing these factors, after a trial of drill and repetition, a series of life situations can be worked out which have or appear to have a direct emotional content for the patient. He can be exposed to traffic situations in the ward or in the home where wheel chairs are being used and can learn the distance he needs to maintain in order to avoid being hit by one of the wheels of other patients or hitting objects in the house. He can be given tools to work with in the shop that permit a choice of relationship to his hands as he works. For example, a series of contacts with the not-too-smooth files used with hand-tooled plastics may assist him in making concentrated efforts at distance judgments. A series of stairs prepared with mats to offset the harm that could come from complete falls can be used to show the distance relationships necessary for climbing or for descending.

In terms of training for right and left, the patients can be permitted to find their own way to the diningroom by a series of left and right directions. The lure of satisfying hunger may prove to be a satisfactory stimulant to learning. A particular planned excursion can be made into the business district and the patient given left and right instructions for a proposed meeting place. If he fails to arrive at the proper place, he may of necessity be stranded. By following the patient, any harm to him through being lost can be obviated. These and other similar methods were used in the army situation and in most cases resulted in a reduction of the disability.

Summary of Receptive Aphasia Therapy

In the preceding pages are shown the specific language problem areas of a receptive nature which may be seen in the brain-injured adult. It should be stressed and repeated, however, that the therapist, in the author's opinion, should possess an organismic viewpoint toward aphasia. The patient should be seen as a whole, a total responding individual, reacting to his environment to the best of his nonintegrated cortical ability. As the patient is first seen and examined and later comes into treatment, he does not present a series of disconnected, separate agnosias. Usually the problem presented is a generalized one of a lack of contact with the communicating world and the various discrete areas of the problem are covered by an over-all façade of frustrated effort to communicate. It is often impossible at an early stage to penetrate this generalized picture and recognize the specific underlying individual agnosias. The total impression of receptive aphasia was described at one time by Halstead and Wepman as "a disturbance of comprehension of spoken or written paragraphs, sentences or phrases. The disturbance is general rather than specific and results in a failure to grasp essential meanings. It is fundamentally a disturbance in pattern or organization of language." [24] These descriptive sentences connote the very difficult and challenging problem that faces the therapist. At the onset of training with the seriously affected patient, a bridge of communication must be established through any means available before therapy can even be attempted.

General Therapeutic Suggestions

First postexamination contacts with the patient should be spent in exploring the many avenues of reception. From the leads given by the examination, it is often possible to limit the direct immediate approach to either an aural or a visual component. Fortunately in almost every case one pathway, visual, aural, or tactile, will be seen to be less seriously impaired than the others. Using this least affected mode, the first contacts may be spent in simple, but psychologically gratifying, problem solving. There appears to be a tremendous effect obtained by setting a problem of any sort that the patient can achieve. The satisfaction obtained may be out of all proportion to the magnitude of the task, but it must be recalled by the therapist that in most cases the patient has been attempting the total act of communication previously and has been consistently frustrated. By undertaking the simple task and obtaining success and closure, approbation, and a kind of silent applause, the patient is made to feel whole, successful, and in contact with his demanding environment, often for the first time. These first attempts need have no relation to the therapeusis planned or foreseen. They are intended as the empathic approach to the patient and should be kept at a constant success level. In almost every case some such success-task can be found in one language modality or another. The following suggestions are not intended as workable approaches to any particular patient, but are illustrations of first tasks that have been used successfully with receptive-aphasic adults.

A patient with a widespread and seriously delimiting receptive problem showed a slightly less impaired ability in visual recognition than in any of the other modes of reception. As a first task, the Dolch picture words were presented to him, one at a time. Since

---

[24] W. C. Halstead and J. M. Wepman, "The Halstead-Wepman Aphasia Screening Test," *Journal of Speech and Hearing,* XIV (March, 1949).

these cards show pictures of easily recognizable common objects, such as a book, a bus, a child, etc., they were felt to be within the recent experience of the patient. Upon presentation no questions were asked. The picture was shown and referred to the actual object present in the room. The response required was indicated by pointing to the picture, then to the object, then to the printed name appearing next to the picture. It was recognized that the printed name was meaningless to the patient, but the fact of its presence was intended and used as requesting its evocation. (This patient had previously shown a letter agnosia on examination where the separate letters were exposed out of context.) On the therapeutic presentation, however, he was able to select the sound made by the first letter of the word after the picture presentation. When this recognition was duly appreciated by the therapist and commented upon, both by word and by expression in response to the patient's questioning looks, an immediate attitude and facial expression of pleasure were observed. (This was the fourth attempt to select a task that would elicit a response in this patient.) With a means of communication established, it was possible through continuous display of these pictures to establish an empathic contact between patient and therapist. By using other related techniques the patient was stimulated to continue various approaches until the separate techniques discussed under the agnosias could be brought into the therapy.

Another patient whose greatest retained ability, although even this mode was seriously affected, was in the aural area responded to the sounds made by various animals and objects. Thus, a picture of a cow elicited no response until the therapist repeated many times the common "moo" sound made by that animal. As the patient learned to associate the sound with the picture or in some instances the sound with a charade-like acting out of the animal or object, she was able to repeat the sound by presentation without previous therapist-produced attempts. These common sounds were then related to graphic phonetic presentations until the sound of a previously described animal could be elicited by the printed word.

Another patient obtained his first success by associating names orally presented with objects of a concrete nature placed in his hand. A hammer which when held by the patient elicited neither action nor language became meaningful and productive of language when the therapist performed a pounding act on an imaginary nail and repeated the symbolic name "hammer." This patient had pretraumatically been a carpenter and developed his first words in the area of his vocation. As an illustration, the first words expressed correctly in addition to the word hammer were "saw," "vise," "brace and bit," and "drill." Simple presentation and repetition, however, were not enough. The patient needed tactual contact before a correct response and the consequent closure could be obtained.

In general the therapist must convey by every means at his disposal, by thought, by word, by action, and by attitude, his desire to be helpful. No matter how simple the task, it must be approached with all seriousness. Patience is probably the greatest necessity of the successful therapist, for progress at the early stage of treatment is difficult to obtain and slow in coming. Learning apparently takes place by complete increments and not by any additive process. When a process is failed and closure is not obtained, the therapist must be alert to the patient's frustration. Simple frustrating signs can usually be overcome by an attitude of urging greater effort. Refusal and rejection, attitudes of withdrawal, overemotionality, and therapist-rejection must be carefully observed and reacted to positively. Shifting to another approach before these reactions assume the positiveness of the catastrophic reaction is an essential. The successful therapist must evaluate the effect of continued perseveration, impulsive and seemingly unrelated behavior, neurological and physical fatigue, and lack of shift. Constant stimulation, helpful suggestions over the parts causing the greatest delay and repetition, being partially helpful but permitting the patient to complete the set task, and exhibiting no great tension while the patient is attempting to respond are all very necessary to the establishment of patient-therapist rapport.

With the establishment of an empathic relationship through some means of communication and consistent achievable success by the patient, it is possible to proceed from these described first steps to the suggestions made earlier on the specific agnosia problems. The receptive aphasias are slow to respond to therapy in the early stages. They frequently resolve themselves more quickly, however, than do the other aphasic problems once some mode is established and first successes are obtained.

Chapter 13

DIRECT THERAPY IN EXPRESSIVE APHASIA

Continuing the direct approaches for reducing the language disturbances of the aphasic adult, the present chapter deals with the expressive forms of the problem. As in the receptive phases discussed earlier, the form of presentation will follow the procedure of discussing the specific expressive areas, called *apraxias,* with a summary devoted to the over-all expressive problem. In addition, the generalized aphasic disturbances called *paraphasia, anomia* and *dysarthria* will be presented, with some of the approaches that have proved useful in reducing their portion of the problem. These latter problems are seen in both receptive and expressive aphasias and always present a particularly difficult obstacle to recovery. For clarity the divisions of the presentation will follow the form of the aphasia examination discussed in Chapter 8.

Apraxia as used in the present context is defined as "loss of ability to execute simple voluntary acts. The loss tends to be specific for elementary units of action in expressing language." [1] The differentiation between the apraxias used in this text refers only to the different types of voluntary acts used in language, for example, the muscular performance involved in grasping or pointing with the hand called *general nonverbal apraxia,* or the muscular act involved in articulating oral speech, called *verbal apraxia.*

Expressive aphasia as an entity is seen as the over-all motor problem involved in communication. It should be borne in mind that the individual exhibiting an aphasia is more than an average human having some degree of difficulty in expressing himself in language. He must be considered as a total organism reacting to the best of his ability in every social contact. Re-education of aphasics from this viewpoint necessitates an approach that is far beyond a training program involving speech and language technique and drill—it involves a constant reorientation of the personality structure. For with each change in the language constructs of the individual he becomes a different organism, reacting to his environ-

---

[1] W. C. Halstead and J. M. Wepman, *Manual for the Aphasia Screening Test* (Chicago: The Authors, 1949).

ment in a different way, with a changed percept of the world as well as a changed ability to communicate with the world. Expressive aphasia re-education, like its counterpart, receptive aphasia training, must encompass the changes necessary to the individual in his new relation to himself and to life.

It is also necessary to remember that aphasic disturbances almost never appear in discrete form. Every expressive aphasic patient exhibits some degree of receptive disability, and conversely receptive aphasic patients are to some degree disabled in the expressive sphere. The approach used should be determined by the phase of the disturbance which seems to be most delimiting to the patient as he comes to therapy. Usually, the facet of the problem which will seem to be of most importance to the therapist will be the most seriously affected area. It must be remembered, however, that this may not be true of the patient's own viewpoint. For example, a patient with a total alexia and only a partial verbal apraxia may be far more concerned with his limited ability to express himself than he is with his total inability to read. Therapy must be adjusted to the needs of the patient at every stage of the re-education or recovery process.

General (Nonverbal) Apraxia

This is the specific inability to perform muscular acts meaningfully and purposively. In the present context the emphasis is placed upon the nonverbal acts concerned in language production. Directly, this concerns the act of grasping a pen or pencil or using the index finger for such acts as directional indicators. Other nonverbal acts are seen in many apraxic patients and frequently are dealt with in therapy in order to relieve the patient of some of his immediate anxiety about his ability to function in society. Such acts may include combing the hair, grasping a toothbrush, or tying the laces of a pair of shoes. The number of these associated acts that are of concern is practically legion. The therapist should be prepared to deal with any or all of them that are expressed as problems by the patient. One patient felt his most serious defect to be his inability to feed himself because of his inability to control the muscles of the hand in such a way as to handle the tableware. It was only after this problem was solved that he was able to bring himself to an acceptance of the total therapeutic process for language.

Training the Grasp.—Therapy for the general apraxias usually is very direct. The task is performed by the therapist. The patient observes the act and attempts to imitate the therapist's performance.

Most often some direct assistance is necessary. The patient's hand is brought into the proper position for grasping a pencil; for example, the therapist holds the patient's hand around the pencil as the act of writing a simple word or phrase is attempted. Often it is necessary to begin with an oversized pencil which makes grasping easier. Sometimes the first grasping act is demonstrated and taught with chalk and the act performed is that of writing on a blackboard in large sweeping motions. When the level of performance aimed at is writing, it has proved most successful to produce words that are meaningful rather than nonsense letters or unattached and meaningless lines. When the task begins with simple grasping rather than as complex a task as writing, it is of importance that the patient understand the purpose of the performance and the goal he is attempting to reach through the undifferentiated exercise.

A useful beginning tool for grasping exercise has been found to be some soft object like a bean-bag which offers less resistance to the grasping act and which permits some degree of hold to be obtained. When simple grasping can be obtained, the picking-grasping-placing act used in such tasks as a simple pegboard have been found to be valuable. The pegboard permits some self-timing and consequent competition with earlier efforts, which may be stimulating to the patient and calls forth greater effort than simple grasping without observable end. Other techniques used include the first acts of grasping a softball, or the handle of a baseball bat of sufficient size to require the gross movements of the hand. A later stage of training may consist of throwing and catching a softball or batting a thrown ball.

After the first grasping act has been achieved by the patient, he should be shifted to the task of grasping successively smaller objects, until holding a pencil or pen becomes easy for him. In the progression to grasping for the act of writing, the common daily grasping acts mentioned above can be taught. In general the early phases of teaching must be by demonstration and by assistance. As these early simple tasks are learned and more complex hand-arm tasks are attempted, the patient should be permitted to try the acts by himself before the therapist assists him. It will be found to be very helpful to begin each therapeutic session with some new common practical act. It has been the author's experience that these simple acts are easily learned and retained. The success obtained by attempting some new task and succeeding at it is extremely beneficial to the general rapport desired. Most frequently it has been observed that patients need instruction in only a few simple tasks in order to regain their former ability but need considerable practice before they regain their former skill.

One of the complicating factors in many apraxic patients is the presence of hemiplegia on the dominant side. When this condition persists, the patient must not only learn to overcome an apraxia but must be trained in skilful performance with his nondominant hand and arm. The latter phase of the problem may be more difficult to overcome than the basic apraxia. Usually this remains a feature of therapy throughout a considerable portion of the therapeusis. There are many levels of apraxia seen, and it is wise usually to begin at the highest level possible for the patient rather than beginning with the most fundamental. Since in communication the act of writing is the most important of the general nonverbal tasks, the patient should be tried at that level first. Only after it is observed that grasping a writing instrument cannot be achieved by the patient should other simpler tasks be attempted. After the grasping and movements of writing can be performed easily and meaningfully by the patient, therapy should continue with the writing act. (See section on "Agraphia," pages 224–26.)

Verbal Apraxia

In the minds of many neurologists, especially the noted English practitioner Wilson, verbal apraxia was synonymous with expressive aphasia. Wilson believed that ". . . on the executive side motor aphasia is a part of apraxia; the patient is not paralyzed but he cannot say what he wants to say, as the apraxic cannot do as he wants to do." [2] This viewpoint is one that restricts aphasia to a mere expression of thought and overlooks the many more complex aspects of the aphasic adult's problem. In the present text the verbal expressive difficulty is considered as one of the specific language defects we are dealing with. It is well represented as Wilson expresses it from the specific consideration of a part of the total problem. The aphasic patient exhibiting a verbal apraxia is delimited in his ability to "say what he wants to say," but this is believed to be part of a generalized complex in which he is also limited in thinking what he wants to think and doing what he wants to do. With his constricted thought processes and his limitations of idea and, as Goldstein holds, his "loss of ability to grasp the essential nature of a process," [3] he is

---

[2] T. Weisenburg and K. McBride, *Aphasia* (New York: The Commonwealth Fund, Division of Publications, 1935), p. 90.

[3] Kurt Goldstein, *Aftereffects of Brain Injuries in War* (New York: Grune & Stratton, Inc., 1942), p. 211.

also unable to express in verbal language form the ideas that he does possess.

The verbal apraxia part of the total problem may seem to outweigh all other parts of the problem, however, for the patient's difficulty in verbal expression is easily the most direct and overt part of the symptomatology. When it is combined with other disabilities on the expressive side of language, it becomes a very delimiting part of the disorder, for man depends to a marked degree upon his ability to state in spoken language his inner feelings, his attitudes, and his thoughts. More often than in any of the other areas of language, the inability to speak becomes a fixation point for the patient, and the other areas seem relatively unimportant to him. Despite this, it is often necessary to approach the verbal apraxia obliquely through the other areas, which may be more approachable and more easily resolved.

Therapy for verbal apraxia has had a longer history than therapy for the other apraxias and agnosias. As has previously been discussed, the therapeutic problem in the aphasias has been for many years considered as a speech problem because of the very nature of the disability, the patient's inability to speak. This very concentration upon the speech act may well be one of the reasons why therapy has progressed as slowly as it has for the aphasic adult, for direct speech approaches are very limiting and hence restricted to this one phase of the greater language defect. It has been the author's experience that verbal apraxia, like the other specific aspects of the aphasic problem, tends to be resolved through approaches and techniques designed to reduce many specific problems other than simple expression. Stated differently, aphasia as a generalized problem reacts to educative and psychological therapies in a nonspecific manner even though the techniques used may be designed to offset a specific phase.

Direct therapy for verbal apraxia as most frequently employed is also a part of the therapy advised for a different aspect of the total problem, namely, the anomias, which will be discussed in a later section as a problem involved in almost every aphasic disorder. The following techniques used to illustrate the direct approach to verbal apraxia will also be found useful in resolution of the anomias.

Training in Speech Sounds.—Where the apraxia is complete, it is often found necessary to begin training at the fundamental phonetic level. If the patient can imitate sounds, the therapist may try to teach some of the phonetic patterns directly. Patients may need to learn the lip sounds *p, b,* and *m* through imitation, using a visual clue. The therapist indicates the position of the lips while seated opposite the patient and asks for an attempted imitation. As the patient closes the lips and opens them he is taught to differentiate between the sounds by the usual speech technique of observing tactually the passage of air through the nose for *m* and the oral escape on *p* and *b*. The latter sounds are differentiated by placing the patient's hand on the therapist's larynx or cheek while the two sounds are produced. The voiced component of the *b* is differentiated in this manner from the unvoiced characteristics of the *p*. It may be found useful in these patients to present the printed letter at the same time as the oral presentation and because of a complicating alexia it may also be found useful to have the patient trace the letters as he sees them on the paper and feels them in contact with the therapist. After these three sounds are recognized from the many clues, the three front vowels may be added. These vowel sounds, *e* as in *even, a* as in *ape* and *ah* as in *are,* can be differentiated by the degree of openness of the mouth. At the same time they can be presented in written form on a blackboard and the patient taught to trace them with chalk and later on paper. By a combination of the three lip consonants and the three front vowels, the idea of vocal production is often obtained by the patient. With little additional encouragement the other sounds often can be added spontaneously by the patient.

The Visualized Consonants.—While the illustrations given refer to only the first stages of recovery from the verbal apraxias, it can be seen that they would need to be elaborated upon and extended for many patients. It is necessary in many cases to develop a large part of the phonetic alphabet before closure is obtained. When this is found to be necessary, the author believes that patients learn most readily the sound patterns for the visualized consonants, the lip-, lip-teeth, and tongue-teeth sounds (*p* as in *Peter, b* as in *brown, m* as in *made, f* as in *full, v* as in *voice, th* as in *thin* and *th* as in *then*). From these easily seen sounds, progression should follow the oral pattern through the front-tongue-palatal sounds of *s, z, sh, l,* and *r*. After these the back-tongue-palatal sounds of *k* and *g* should be used, and finally, if necessary, the more complex combinations of *ch* and *j* as well as the middle *zh* and final *ng*. It has been the author's good fortune that in none of the patients seen over the past fifteen years has it been necessary to teach beyond the middle of the second category. Most often, when interest can be maintained through simple sound presentation, a reiteration of the first category until mastered has been found sufficient for teaching at this phonetic level.

First Use of Words.—One patient whose problem was not complicated by an alexia of great proportions found it much easier to work on the phonetic approach when the examples used were combined immediately into short meaningful words. Thus single-syllable words like *map, bomb,* etc., were analyzed phonetically in writing and illustrated by pictures. These words were then demonstrated by single phonetic sound presentation in the manner described above until the patient grasped the construct of sound production as being meaningful and within his capacity.

From these simple direct approaches to the apraxia, the therapy can usually progress to a naming game, where the common objects in the environment that have simple names are analyzed and used as illustrative material. Through this second stage the problem of the anomia and the apraxia can be approached simultaneously. Where verbal apraxia is present, it most often must be the direct point of beginning therapy, even though it is not approached. For example, when a patient either cannot make a start in the manner suggested or cannot be stimulated to try such simple material or even when he does try but cannot maintain interest, it may be necessary to seek out an avenue that gives him a more direct interest. When the history indicates a particular vocational or avocational interest of the patient, all approaches may need to be developed within that interest area.

Progressing beyond teaching the meaning of sounds and relating them to particular phonetic patterns most often means beginning language at the single-word nominative level of speech. At this stage the patient has mastered or retained the ability to produce single sounds or syllables upon request. Most often he is unable to produce them voluntarily without stimulation. Even though this stage has not been achieved, in the interest of progress it is best to go on to word-naming as soon as possible. Teaching the ability to recognize the symbolic nature of language attached to the singly presented object or picture may be a part of the therapeusis for a considerable portion of the early stage of therapy. That is, word-naming or the disability in that area called *anomia* may be a symptom as persistent as is seen in the verbal apraxic adult's entire recovery. It should be approached early and worked on consistently through the training process. Until words can be attached with meaning to objects, the free flow of meaningful language will always be defective and the patient seriously handicapped.

The most common technique used in this area and one that seems to be as simple and direct as possible is the presentation of single objects or pictures and establishment of as many language clues as possible to the presentation. For example, a picture of a baby, accompanied by the printed word "baby" and the spoken word, is presented without requesting a response from the patient. A series of three or four such stimulus-groups is shown. Upon second presentation the patient is requested to repeat the word after the therapist or to try copying the printed word. On the third presentation the word is not spoken and the patient is merely shown the picture and the accompanying printed word and asked to supply the spoken word. If this is unsuccessful, the printed word is withheld, the picture is presented, the spoken word is supplied, and the patient is asked to supply the written word. On later presentations, the picture is presented with a group of other pictures, the word is spoken or presented in written form, and the patient is asked to select the correct picture; or the picture is presented, neither a printed nor an oral clue is given, and the patient is asked to speak or write the name.

As many variations of this technique as possible may need to be used. Certain stimulus-words may fail to elicit a worth-while response. To maintain interest, different stimulus-words must be used with the caution that there must be enough repetition of the first pictures to enable the factor of repetition to take effect. Even with some success, considerable training and repetition may be necessary until the principle of names for pictured objects is comprehended by the patient. In some cases picture presentation with the printed word may be worthless. The alexic patient finds the printed word as difficult to recognize as he does the oral word pattern. For these patients, oral word presentation with the picture may be as far as one is able to go. In still other cases it may be necessary to teach sight recognition of the printed word with the picture, since a complicating factor may be an auditory agnosia. The particular approach will of course be limited by various additional facets of the problem.

Using Material of Interest to the Patient.—Rapport and co-operation of the patient correlates very highly in therapy with the therapist's ability to keep the material on an acceptable level of interest for the patient. The therapist must always be alert to the problem of patient fatigue, and this factor seems to be at its highest when the material used fails to stimulate the patient to continued effort. To illustrate this, a particular patient who consistently failed to make progress at the initial stages of therapy responded with seeming alacrity to the same level of therapy when it was adjusted to his pretraumatic vocational interest of music. First words were obtained through the use of such word illustrations as sharps and flats pictured and spoken and names of musical instruments, such as *piano, flute, violin, drum,* etc. While the phonetic analysis was far more difficult for this patient, he obtained a rapid series of insights once the idea of spoken language became integrated through these fairly complex sound patterns.

As has previously been indicated, one of the most difficult parts of all therapy for aphasic adults is the problem of suitable material. The author and his staff searched for many months and still continue to search for material that will be generally useful for the aphasic adult. Material usually must be developed separately for almost every aphasic patient during therapy. Material which has proved useful for one patient may be of no use at all for another, even though the phase of the problem being treated seems to be the same. One of the therapist's most difficult tasks may be this development of material that is useful with the individual patient. Throughout the early stages of therapy this problem often remains constantly before the therapist and requires a constant alertness to the patient's needs and interests.

Where interest is difficult to obtain and to maintain, it may be necessary to seek out the area of greatest pretraumatic interest for the patient and develop a naming vocabulary in that area before approaching the common nouns of the current environment. The therapist may find that it is necessary to develop a knowledge of many areas which previously had been of only passing, if of any, interest to him. For this reason one therapist may become expert in astronomy and another may need to be learned in the language of classical music. The author recalls an instance in which it was necessary for him to develop a personal vocabulary dealing with law and legal terminology before he had succeeded in reaching the patient on even the simplest approach to language.

This very need for reaching the patient on his interest level in vocabulary makes the treatment and the training of the aphasic adult the fascinating problem that it is. It keeps the therapist constantly on the alert intellectually and the therapy does not resolve itself into a series of simple repetitive drills and exercises. In fact while the breakdown of techniques which have proved successful or useful in past therapies may seem dull and repetitive, the actual practice of developing material and seeking self-knowledge that will appeal to the patient has proved so stimulating that many therapists thrown into this field without previous interest have become excellent aphasia therapists.

Using Tactual Stimuli.—Verbal apraxias may also present a continuing problem when they do not or cannot be reached through aural or visual stimuli. In the author's experience two cases needed to be approached with tactual stimuli from the very beginning. In these patients it was necessary to use objects which could be handled and names were attached to these objects in a functional manner rather than through the commonly accepted symbolic approach. For example, a hammer made a particular sound as it struck a metal bell; an automobile, a toy one in this case, made a unique sound as it rolled across a table, or paper as it was torn made a sound which could be differentiated from other sounds. Using these and other onomato-poetic patterns, these patients were taught to imitate the sounds being made by the various materials being presented. Through continuous presentation the symbolic nature of the sound relating to the object was recognized through the conditioning process and from this, the sound made by humans was an easy step. (The easiness of this step is seen only in retrospect, since the time element involved extended over a month.) After sound relations of this nature had been perceived and recognized by the patients, the phonetic approach discussed above was used until simple words could be formed and attached to objects. This is by all odds the most roundabout direct approach developed, yet apparently it was necessary, for nothing else attempted seemed to be of any value in reducing the disorder for these particular patients.

Raising the Level of Language.—From the word-naming level most patients need almost an equal amount of time spent on the "use" level of language. Learning seemed to follow the same pattern that the development of speech in children follows. First-learned words are invariably nouns, followed by verbs, adjectives, and then adverbs. While the first group, the nouns, seem to be learned in isolated and separate fashion and the second group also, at least to some degree, the last two groups seem to come in mixed fashion. Thus, a patient may be on the naming level for some time, and, while able to increase his vocabulary of names with some degree of spontaneity, he will still be unable to add any words in terms of use (or on the verb level) without a comparatively long training period. Usually after the naming level has been established to some degree the therapist should try to shift to the verb level. Thus, a ball which can be named should be shown in use as a bouncing ball, or a thrown ball; a man walks or runs, sits or lies down; a dog barks; etc. By testing this level at various times, the therapist finds the time when the patient seems to be able to go beyond simple naming.

With the development of the verb level of language the therapist can also work on the formation of the simple sentence. These simple sentences should be composed of noun and verb only at first. Lack of use of prepositions, adjectives, and other parts of speech should be ignored. In fact, in teaching it is found that most ideas can be expressed rather well in short two- or three-word sentences. Following the beginning of sentences, it will be found to be of considerable value in many patients to go back to the pronoun forms. Patients of even moderate education have a ready recognition level for the personal pronouns, and the very egocentricity of their problems makes it easy to show the value of "I" and "we" and from these the rest of the common personal pronouns. After short sentences can be made, even though with some effort, some patients respond most rapidly if that form is insisted upon at least during the direct therapeutic sessions. As the patient adds verbs to his nouns, the adjectives can be added rather simply. A ball now becomes a round ball, or a tall man is differentiated from a short man.

At this stage it is frequently found that the patient retains a sense of likeness and oppositeness. When this is found, voluntary language can be stimulated by the therapist's suggesting the use of a particular word through the use of its opposite and through an analogue. For example, if the desired word is "sun" it can be obtained by the therapist's saying "moon" in a sentence which answers the question "What gives light in the daytime?" If no answer is forthcoming the therapist can continue the question by asking, "Is it the moon?" This evoking of voluntary language through additional language clues may play an important part in early therapy and may be of great assistance in giving the patient the necessary method of thinking about speech for him to produce his own voluntary language attempts. Sentence completion and word selection by multiple choice in a printed form are frequently used devices at this stage of training.

In concluding these remarks on the verbal apraxias and the direct therapies that seem to be most useful in beginning their resolution, it should be stressed that the illustrations used are merely meant to be suggestive of the approach that may be necessary for individual patients. The therapist must constantly be alert to the stage of treatment that the patient needs for his expression at that time. This constantly changes, whether through a cumulative learning process or through a series of new or relearned Gestalts. Staying ahead of the patient and keeping him constantly stimulated and slightly frustrated so that he will continue to show growth and change may challenge the ingenuity of even the best and most experienced therapist. It is certainly true in this area, probably more than any other, that old therapeutic or educative skills may be of little value and may have to be discarded in terms of the patient's needs and the rate of his change and growth. Staying at a stage of development too long may succeed only in satisfying the patient and in plateauing his learning curve. If this continues for any length of time, the patient's response level may become routinized and he may stand still for a considerable period and require an extended therapeutic effort to move ahead again. The patient showing a verbal apraxia needs to be stimulated toward a single goal—free voluntary expression. Any stage below that level must be considered a stage in development only. (For additional techniques see Goldstein's chapter on therapy in his *After-effects of Brain Injuries in War* and Granich's *Aphasia: A Guide to Retraining.*[4])

Writing Apraxia (Agraphia)

Among the expressive disabilities, the difficulty many aphasic patients have in the sphere of writing is probably next to that of difficulty with free verbalization in its debilitating effect upon the individual. While this varies with the patient according to his needs, everyone, especially the individual who cannot speak, feels that the inability to write is a severe problem. The therapist, too, will find the patient exhibiting an agraphia as a part of his symptom complex an especially complicated therapeutic problem. When the writing capacity is retained, it serves as an excellent choice in place of speech for conveying the patient's thoughts to the therapist. When the ability to write is defective, however, no easy medium is at hand and communication becomes a complex and difficult task. It is unfortunate that in many instances the expressive aphasic adult shows an equal difficulty in both oral and graphic expression.

Therapeutic Approach.—The writing disorder usually takes one of two forms, or perhaps two varying degrees of the same apraxic

---

[4] L. Granich, *Aphasia: A Guide to Retraining* (New York: Grune & Stratton, Inc., 1947).

problem. In terms of the therapy needed, this difference can be considered as a real dichotomy, for the approach is different in the two types of problem. Agraphia is most commonly seen in the patient as a disability in which the individual cannot recall how to formulate the words or letters of the language in cursive script. In the more unusual type, the patient cannot recall how to coordinate the muscles necessary to make the movements of the writing act. The latter type is usually associated with the more generalized nonverbal apraxia mentioned earlier. An additional complicating factor in many aphasic patients is the dominant hemiplegia that accompanies the disorder. When this factor is present, the patient must not only relearn the act of writing in a cortical sense but must also learn to coordinate the activity of the nondominant extremity in a peripheral sense. In general it should be remembered that the approach to the writing skill should accompany other therapy. When it is part of a total therapeutic program, it will ordinarily be found that the writing act will be relearned more rapidly at the early stage of training than will the oral skill of speaking. Since it usually precedes the act of speech, it can in its later stages become a definite part of the training aimed at reducing the verbal disability and can be discontinued as a separate training goal.

First Steps in Training.—For the patient whose disability extends to muscular coordination, the first steps are usually those discussed previously under the general nonverbal apraxias. The patient must be taught how to grasp the writing tool and then how to make the coordinating muscular movements of writing. After the first of these stages is learned, the second is usually accomplished most easily by using chalk on a blackboard. The therapist inscribes printed letters on the board, each letter approximately three to four inches high. Standing behind the patient and grasping his hand, which contains the chalk, the therapist guides the patient's movements through the task of tracing the letters. The movements should at first be straight lines following the printed forms of the letters, to teach the sweep of the arm for major muscular movements. The letters should be called out by the therapist as they are drawn by the patient. It will be found helpful if all the letters of the alphabet in both written and printed form appear at the top of the blackboard for reference by the patient and the therapist. Where the patient does not know the alphabet, even in a serial fashion, some initial instruction in locating the different letters of the alphabet should be tried, even though it is not imitated by the patient. This can be done by simply repeating the alphabet, either *in toto* or in five-letter groups. It was not found useful to teach the patients the alphabet by rote.

After the patient recognizes the tracing act and can select letters as they are called to him, he should be permitted to copy letters by name from the examples given on the board. If necessary, the therapist should continue to guide the patient's hand and arm through the movements of writing. Following some success at this stage, the patient should repeat the act with script rather than the printed form. This should still be done at the blackboard and should still be with the large letter-forms given separately. Guiding the hand and arm should be kept at a minimum, but should be used as much as is necessary. No attempt at attaining a high degree of accuracy need be made. While accurate and highly legible writing is a part of the goal, it becomes a matter of concern, if at all, in later stages of training.

Writing at the Desk.—After the act can be performed with single cursive letters at the blackboard, the work should shift to writing at the desk. Where the patient is hemiplegic it is best to start training the left hand immediately, even though it seems indicated that the right hand will eventually return to function. This latter process is such a long one that writing will be well incorporated and useful to the patient with the left hand long before the function in the right hand is restored. In beginning work on paper, it is found useful to start with large print on paper lined at every two inches. The patient's attempts should first be printed and then script again. There may be some very necessary periods of hand- and arm-guidance at this stage just as there was at the earlier stage. In this period the patient should be seated with the therapist standing above him but to the rear, reaching over his shoulder and grasping his hand. It is sometimes found necessary to begin again with tracing, then progressing to copying and finally to writing from oral stimuli. At times a good exercise is to present printed material and ask the patient to copy it in script. The large print and script should be used until a free-flowing movement can be made, with progress to words as soon as possible.

In combined therapy when verbal training is being given, it is found useful to reinforce the words being attempted orally with the written forms. As the movements become easier, the size of the practice can be reduced progressively until the normal or usual size of script is being used.

After the beginning stages of writing have been mastered, such practice texts as Gardner's *Left Handed Writing*[5] have been found to be useful for patients who need to shift to the left hand. For those patients who are not being shifted, the texts found most helpful were *Correlated Handwriting: Practice Books 1, 2 and 3.*[6] Writing practice should continue throughout therapy as a part of the training program, but as has already been mentioned it should only be given direct attention until the act can be mastered on a functional basis and then should be used as a tool for assisting the remainder of therapy. Because it is so useful to the other language techniques, it should be approached as soon as possible in the training program. This should be emphasized even to the point of delaying some of the more severely affected areas.

Number Apraxia

As was seen earlier in the two-level consideration of general apraxia and agraphia, there are two levels of numerical disability definable in the aphasic patient. The first of these is the low-level disability in which the patient is unable to use numbers in any form. Even when he is able to recognize numbers, the patient may be unable to speak or write the number forms. At this level the dysfunction is recognized as the patient fails to count or to write the digital series successfully. While this disability is of most concern in calculation (see page 229), it is of greater importance to the patient in the everyday acts of life. These patients cannot produce their addresses, telephone numbers, or other identifying numbers with accuracy. To the nonaphasic patient this may seem like a rarely used and easily overlooked ability. Because of the very simplicity of the acts involved, however, it becomes an exceedingly frustrating problem to the patient. The correct recalling of dates, the number of the ward in the hospital in which one lives, and the number of one's possessions all are facts which may be needed and used daily. The inability to produce them voluntarily is often found to be both debilitating and frustrating.

Combining Number Training with Other Therapies.—Direct therapy for the number apraxias can become a part of the training suggested earlier for agraphia. The patient can learn to copy or

---

[5] Warren Gardner, *Left Handed Writing* (Danville, Ill.: Interstate Press, 1945).
[6] Frank Freeman, *Correlated Handwriting: Practice Books 1, 2, and 3* (Columbus, O.: Zaner-Bloser Co., 1927–1931).

to trace the number series from 1 to 10. Imitation of the written form can be accompanied by verbal repetition of the written number. Serial counting is sometimes retained even when the number-production sense is disturbed; if so serial numbers can be used in the therapeutic process. Associating the numbers as they are counted with objects or items being named in training for the verbal apraxias is a useful approach. Ordinarily, it has been found most successful to combine number training with other expressive acts during the early stages of training rather than to treat it in an isolated fashion.

The material for number training is available everywhere. A patient appears to learn most rapidly when numbers are used whenever it is practical to use them. One patient found that counting and writing the number attached to body parts assisted him in recapturing a body image. For this patient a drawing of a human being was used. As he named the parts of the body, he was asked to ascribe numbers to each part. In this fashion the nose became number 1, the mouth number 2, the eyes numbers 3 and 4, the ears numbers 5 and 6, etc. Later, the patient was able to count the nose as one, the mouth as one, the ears as two, the feet as two, the fingers as five on the right and five on the left. Through this procedure both names and numbers became familiar to him.

Another patient whose previous interest lay in painting and in form delineation learned both language and numbers at an early stage by identifying the colors used on a series of pictures and attaching a number to each color as he saw and produced in both writing and speech the color name. A third patient learned numbers by identifying the tools used in a work situation in occupational therapy. It was made his task among others to be responsible for the tools used. This was a link with his past, for as a workman he needed to do the same thing. As he replaced his tools in his workbox he was asked to recall the name and to count each tool. The hammer became number 1, the files numbers 2, 3, and 4, etc. Later, he was asked to check these numbers and names against a printed list and to write down the name and number of each object.

A word of caution is entered here. The therapist must be careful not to delay the training in number production until the other apraxic areas are well along in recovery. When this is done and the patient must return to simple fundamentals again, it may serve to discourage him and to delay the entire recovery process. Likewise, the early stages of training for all the seriously affected apraxic difficulties may well need to be very fundamental. It is not difficult at this early stage to stimulate the patient in many directions at the same level. Using numbers as a means of identification and as an additional means of association for the learning of names and practice in writing serves to resolve two problems at one time.

In analysis of the aphasic problem it may appear that the ability to verbalize any symbolic meaningful word or to write any purposive expression will extend into the area of numbers. By and large this has not proved to be the case clinically. Many patients find number expression easy when verbalizations are impossible; others recover rapidly in number production while verbalization in general lags far behind. Still other patients regain considerable language before numbers become meaningful at all. Since this separate function of numbers in communication has been recognized, its corollary has been also perceived. Training in the use of numbers serves to reduce the dysfunction in that area. Apparently it does not, however, serve to reduce the disability noticed in any other communication area.

Calculation Apraxia (Acalculia)

This is the higher level disability in use of numbers. Aphasic patients in whom it is detected that the lower level number apraxia is present will invariably show a marked defect in calculating ability. The converse of this is not true, however. Many patients show a retained number-production ability without the more complex retention of use of numbers in a mathematical sense. Within the broad range of activities covered by acalculia, the simplest levels may be affected separately from the higher mathematical functions. Some patients can use numbers mathematically for simple problems like the making of change or selecting the correct amount for the purchase of small articles, especially when these purchases fall within the smaller number series up to twenty-five, but experience great difficulty in using numbers for nonconcrete mathematical abstractions like addition, subtraction, multiplication, and division. Most frequently, however, there is seen a more extensive problem where the use of numbers in calculation is completely absent. As mentioned earlier, the tendency for the number faculty to coexist with other verbal forms is great. It is noted in most patients, however, that the two difficulties, verbal apraxia and calculation apraxia, do not interact to the point that they are resolved simultaneously. Resolution of each area seems to follow direct training in that area, and there seems to be little transfer effect between the two.

While it has been found practical to work simultaneous problems in lower level number apraxia with the beginning stages of treatment for the other apraxias, the same is not true of the higher levels. Calculation therapy, it has been found, needs to be approached separately and not intermixed with training for verbalization, writing, or general apraxia. At the same time the therapist should consider devoting a considerable portion of the therapy to the area of calculation when the patient expresses a need for the ability. This may occur early in therapy in some patients or may never arise as a directly expressed need. In the latter instance, the patient's lack of initiative and his generally sheltered life should be taken into consideration and a need stimulated through therapy. This is often necessary for the patient whose activity spheres are limited. As to when it should be taught, the therapist must think of the total progression of the patient in the recovery process. When the patient is about to make contacts outside the home and classroom, numbers become more and more important to him. Before that time he should have started training in this area. The extent of training is completely an individual problem. Some patients express an interest in mathematics through arithmetic, fractions, algebra, and even geometry. The therapist need have little concern about his own competence in the various advanced fields, however. Advanced therapies are easily followed in textbooks, and most patients can progress with little or no help from the therapist once the subject is introduced to them and they can express themselves at the fundamental level. Usually where higher levels are desired it will be found that overcoming the concrete attitudes of the brain-injured and proceeding to an abstract level may be the most frustrating part of the therapy. When the patient can assume an abstract frame of reference, recovery in high level acalculia will not seem difficult.[7]

Construction Apraxia

This is a high level disability growing out of the basic general nonverbal apraxia. The patient exhibits an inability to produce complex figures in drawing or is unable to use the hands for a planned activity beyond the simple grasping and movement controls discussed earlier. The inability to plan action and to perform detailed work is frequently seen when the lower level of coordinate activity is retained. The problem is of course especially delimiting

---

[7] For reference to the techniques needed, see Grace Fernald, *Remedial Techniques in Basic School Subjects* (New York: McGraw-Hill Book Co., Inc., 1943), chap. xiv, or secure any set of mathematical workbooks used in the public schools.

to the patient whose pretraumatic history indicates interest in performance or vocations requiring handwork. There is little direct relation of this disability to the language act, and it needs to be considered by the therapist only when the problem presents itself in therapy through the patient's frustration or indication of concern. When the problem is encountered, it is usually necessary to consider the entire area of nonverbal apraxia. Construction apraxia should receive attention and effort only after the simpler apraxias have been resolved.

In direct therapy it has been found useful to call upon the skills and training of the occupational therapist for assistance with these cases. The tasks set in this area can begin with manual arts that are easy to achieve, planned originally by the therapist. In the hospital aphasia center discussed in an earlier section, the patients were given simple tasks relating to their interests, such as plastic and metal work. Care was used to keep the initial tasks well within the patient's performance ability or, where that was impossible, at the simplest feasible level. A great deal of guidance and assistance was offered. In many instances these occupational tasks were the areas that could be approached first, and language training accompanied the manual efforts. In one patient whose drives were all in the direction of handwork, simple leather-weaving, using many colors, was the original stimulus for securing rapport and cooperation. Through the process of weaving with multicolored leather it was possible to begin teaching the names of the colors and the words describing the movements used, such as *up, over, under, down,* etc. From this verbal accompaniment a beginning was made toward the resolution of the verbal apraxia. The general approach used in training for the construction apraxias was to devote considerable time and effort to them when they were of apparent importance to the patient or when it was necessary to use them to stimulate the patient who otherwise could not accept the more intellectualized verbal acts.

Any task leading to a completion and to closure for the patient seems to be worth while as a starting point. The work should ordinarily proceed from simple gross movements to the finer complex skills. Progression through a series does not seem to be very important in this area. As the patient finds himself able to perform the undifferentiated tasks, self-selection of further activity seems to be most successful as a means of determining what should follow.

To illustrate the relation of construction apraxia to language, one patient, a housewife of fifty-five, showed little improvement in her use of language after many sessions of therapy. By analysis of her frustrations it became apparent that her previous abilities and interests lay in the kitchen rather than in speech or other language acts. By assisting her in the baking of a cake, by showing her how to begin the various acts of sifting flour, rolling dough, measuring quantities of ingredients, and regulating an oven, the therapist was able to make a beginning toward reading, writing, and speech. Flexibility of approach is probably the greatest necessity of the aphasia therapist, and working through such off-the-subject areas as construction and complex muscular movements may be the key to successful therapy in many instances.[8]

Ideokinetic Apraxia

The inability to perform a given task from an oral clue or a non-verbal visual clue is one of the more complex and yet one of the more debilitating of the aphasic patient's problems. When the patient is unable to write the name of a presented object or is unable to carry through a task when it is requested of him, he often seems more frustrated than he does in the more serious debility of being unable to speak. The typical impulsiveness and sometimes the catastrophic reaction patterns of the brain-injured adult are often brought to light in this area. Unlike the agraphic patient, who is basically unable to write, these patients can use graphic skills from either dictation or the visually presented word, but they are unable to express in writing the name of an object presented to them. The idea represented by an object or its translation into a written symbol seems to be disturbed. At another level, even self-ideation or recall of visual memories cannot be expressed because of this failure at relating the thought to the required task. In the predominantly expressive aphasic patient where the inability to perform a particular task is recognized by the patient, the tendency toward affective reaction is often very marked.

Therapeutically, this problem is faced only when the patient indicates a need for such self-expression in the early stages of therapy. Treatment of it has been delayed in most therapeusis largely because of the difficulty of attacking it. When, however, the patient shows the emotional reaction described, the therapist may have to disregard many of the other areas to devise ways and means of overcoming this affect-producing disability. Probably no single area of the aphasia

---

[8] For techniques useful in reducing construction apraxias, see the references cited in Chapter 10, footnote 2, page 139.

problem has proved to be more frustrating to the author. Different approaches have been attempted with a variety of patients, but little or no general approach has proved satisfactory enough to be considered as a technique capable of approaching the problem in a simple way. If a generalization can be made from all the attempted techniques, it would fall into the simple conditioning and even rote-training area. At least, some patients seem to overcome their difficulty in this area at the time that they are working on drill and rote learning through imitation. Showing a picture, writing its name for the patient, repeating the name, having the patient repeat the name in imitation, having the patient copy the written name, etc., repeated many times over, seems to have had some effect that resulted in later learning.

In most instances, however, while the patient did seem to learn to perform ideokinetically, the first demonstrations of his ability seemed to come in examples that had not been used in the therapeusis. For example, one patient was given considerable drill of the type named. The illustrations used were of simple common objects such as a book, a baby, a boy, etc. After a discouraging period of time spent in drill and imitation, the patient wrote the word "dictionary" upon accidentally seeing such a volume on the therapist's desk. He was, however, unable to write the words used as examples for many weeks after this successful performance. Another patient, whose apraxic problem was complicated by a body agnosia, could not point to any given part of the body, both because he did not recall the body image and because the ideokinetic act of pointing was beyond his ability. These two problems were at first approached simultaneously. The body image was shown in an illustration, and rote learning of the parts was used in attempting to reduce that part of the problem. Pointing was illustrated and discussed at some length. The agnosia was resolved through rote drill by therapist indication of the parts of the body and what appeared to be a memorization process of the patient's. Pointing, however, remained unresolved. On one occasion the patient was inadvertently asked to indicate the location of a disrupting noise and he responded by pointing in the general direction from which the noise emanated. Building on this apparently automatic response, the ideokinetic area was explored and eventually resolved.

In all aphasia re-education and therapy, this principle of knowing what the particular stimulus or material may be that succeeds in creating the insights necessary for learning is a difficult one to determine. So much is this true that the author hesitates very

markedly in presenting any of the illustrations used as being indica-
tive of a proper or correct method for the resolution of any facet
of the problems presented.

Summary of the Apraxias

The foregoing sections on the apraxias cover many separate
facets of the expressive aphasic problem. As was seen on the receptive side, however, it is extremely difficult to fractionate the over-
all problem in the individual patient. The patient reacts as a whole.
He does not show isolated specific disorders in his general behavior
pattern. Isolation of the different apraxic areas is a function of the
examination and is used to determine the various pathways that need
to be used to approach the total person.

As the examination form (page 132) indicates, there is a considerable and complicating task of analysis presented in determining
the extent to which any response made by the patient is etiologically
based upon a particular apraxic or agnostic function. Differentiating
the apraxias is a practical device. Re-educating the aphasic patient is
a problem of determining the areas of defect and in consequence the
areas of retained ability for the selection of the most likely avenue
of approach. As has been seen in the discussion of therapy, it is
very rare that a particular apraxic area will be approached from the
viewpoint of that area only. Actually in practice every exercise,
every contact is aimed at the over-all goal of reduction of aphasia,
defined as the generalized "disturbance of expression of well-formed
paragraphs, sentences, or phrases in speech or composition . . .
when complete [it] may result in a total inability of the individual
to express himself in speech or writing. It is fundamentally a disturbance in pattern or organization of language." [9]

Beyond this direct language consideration of the aphasia itself
lies the therapeutic goal of rehabilitation and readjustment of the
individual exhibiting the aphasia. The expressive aphasic patient
cannot speak or write. As a result of this inability at expression in
a common language form he finds it difficult to relate to other humans,
he withdraws and becomes seclusive in his behavior, and he tends to
be irritable and seems at times to be asocial. Further, it must be
recalled that brain injury or disease tends to produce typical behavioral activity as a direct result of the changed neurological entity.
The patient perseverates in language and thought, he reacts impulsively at times and even in a catastrophic manner to many seemingly

[9] Halstead and Wepman, op. cit.

simple frustrating experiences. These and many other behavioral indications make the treatment process as much a psychotherapeutic one as a pedagogic one. This seems to be much more true of the expressive patient than of the receptive for one rather basic reason.

The patient showing an expressive aphasia recognizes his own errors but is impotent to change or correct his faulty efforts. His reactions to self are consequently more definite and overt, his frustrations more evident and more realistic. The therapist must be prepared to offer the supportive therapy that is necessary to stimulate the patient to change. Insights into one's own limitations, the prognosis and the expectations of therapy, are important to the expressive aphasic adult. The lack of self-criticism in the receptive aphasic adult makes this need far less apparent and far less important to him. At the same time the presence of this ability to criticize one's own behavior is one of the important factors in the recoverability of the language processes. It permits self-comparisons, discriminations of behavior, and the possibility of inter-patient comparisons which are exceedingly helpful in therapeusis.

A second and equally important differentiation between the predominantly expressive aphasic patient and the one whose disabilities are largely in the receptive language areas is the former's ability to follow direct stimulation, intelligently and meaningfully. The ability to understand verbal and written instruction makes both the therapy and the pedagogy a more direct and more satisfying process. Materials are more easily secured, and rapport is more easily achieved. Frustrations can be dealt with directly and insights achieved through direct perception. For these reasons and others, the expressive aphasic patient has been found to be the more easily trained, the more satisfactorily treated.

Just as with the receptive aphasias, however, the problems involved cannot be perceived as being the total of a group of separate apraxic difficulties. The expressive aphasic adult must be treated as a patient presenting language and personality inadequacies which frustrate him totally in every walk of life. While treatment can be designed for the individual areas, the results are usually measurable for the patient only in terms of his generalized reaction. The inability to call a particular familiar object by name as he desires to, or as he previously was able to, may be completely frustrating to him even though through therapy he is able to read and to write. The extent of the problem in the patient's mind may well be out of all proportion to the measurable severity or extent of the aphasia. It is important to approach the patient from this total viewpoint, to provide outlets in every area in which he expresses concern, even though by test or observation all the areas do not seem to be of equal importance. It should be axiomatic in treatment for the expressive aphasic patient that the patient sets the goals, the patient sets the pace, and the patient achieves the result. The therapist must serve as teacher and psychologist. He must work toward the goals of language recovery and self-acceptance. Techniques are only of value in an *adjusted individual*. The patient able to speak but unable to adjust will find speaking unimportant.

Anomia

Most consistent of all the language symptoms seen in aphasic patients is the difficulty in naming that appears in almost all patients. This inability to symbolize, to use common names for articles or objects or persons, is so widespread that many authors have classified patients showing it to a marked degree as a separate type of aphasic. Head, the prominent English neurologist, saw this particular symptom as running through the entire aphasia problem and based his theory of aphasia as a disorder of symbolization upon the evident disability represented by the patient's difficulty in translating thought and action into symbolic form.[10]

Naming incapacity is seen in both receptive and expressive types of aphasic adults as described in the present manuscript. The disorder in its purest form is the patient's inability to use common names for the parts of his environment that he wishes to talk about. For instance, upon presentation of a common object like a *fork,* the patient may respond with (*a*) a word which sounds like the name *fork,* such as *pork* or *fort* or *nook;* (*b*) a word which is related to the function of the object, such as *knife* or *spoon;* (*c*) a word which is totally unrelated, like *dog, man,* or any other word; (*d*) no word at all. The prevalence of responses in the first two categories is usually found in the expressive aphasic patient, while the last two types are most often seen in the predominantly receptive patient. These are not arbitrary distinctions, however, and either type of aphasic patient may respond in any of the four ways mentioned. What is more commonly seen is that the expressive type of patient will be able to recognize his errors and will keep on trying to select the correct word, while the receptive patient usually tries a name and gives up after one abortive effort, questioning the therapist as to its cor-

---

[10] Henry Head, *Aphasia and Kindred Disorders of Speech,* 2 vols. (New York: The Macmillan Co., 1926), Vol. I, p. 123.

rectness; or he may try a time or two to get a word out and then give up. This follows the previously discussed ability of these two types of patients in their general capacity for self-criticism.

Anomia Without Other Disability.—The inability to use names in speech may not seem too debilitating until one attempts to get along without nouns, even though the rest of speech is retained. One patient who showed the very rare problem of almost a total anomia without other speech or language defect illustrates this problem very well. This patient from his history sustained a head injury which left him, in the immediate posttraumatic state, a severe expressive aphasic patient. Without training, his generalized aphasia resolved itself within the first four posttraumatic months. He had little or no sensory involvement at any time and after the initial period could read, write, use figures, and talk without difficulty. He could not (and cannot) use names voluntarily. An example of his difficulty is seen in the following verbatim quotation of one of his efforts at description. The presenting problem was to write a description of a picture of a dining alcove with a table set for dinner. He was asked to describe what he saw, leaving blank any word that he could not express.

This is a ———— in the center on it is a thing that keeps what it is made out of from getting lumpy or dirty. Where this meets with the other part is a ————. This is where what they drink is made in. Around it is where you would sit while you ate. To one side is a ———— that holds many things. On the bottom is what would make ———— dark. Also something that would hold what you would make in the thing in the center of the ———— only in this it would be cold. On the top of this is a certain kind of a thing that allows you to see in the dark.

The circumlocutions necessary to express his ideas, the futility that develops from attempts to get meaning into the act of description, and the failure of closure that is so evident in the sample shown have led to a psychological withdrawal from speech and from society. This particular patient, it is believed, has become neurotic as the result of his language incapacity despite the fact that his aphasic manifestation is limited to the area of naming. Unfortunately the patient has shown little or no improvement as this is written, and it is at present conceived as a necessity to use extraordinary means to free him from his secondary psychological confusion and growing maladjustment.

Fortunately this type of problem is rare. The more common type is the anomia which exists as a part of a generalized aphasia.

Usually the inability to use names is a part of a widespread inability to speak and can be resolved in the course of over-all therapy. Many patients, however, while they show a general resolution of their language problems, will show a residual in terms of speed of speech and of word-finding and it is not uncommon to find partial residuals in anomia many years after the onset of the disorder.

Early Therapeusis.—Therapeutically, treatment for anomia should begin with the first contacts with the patient. Therapy for all types of aphasia where speech is the area to be approached most intensely should begin with the naming process. It has been noted that speech recovery in the aphasic adult appears to follow somewhat the same order as does speech development in the child. In both developmental areas of language it is noted that names for objects develop first, followed by action words and then by descriptive or delimiting word forms. Grammatically the order is usually nouns, verbs, adjectives, and adverbs, leading to language in the presyntax stage. Sentences are usually developed in their complete form only after these individual and meaningful words can be used with some degree of ease. Consequently, the first steps in training should be in the area of names or nouns.

For the child and for the adult, it is found useful to use names for objects that are common to daily experience. The child starts to learn words that give him daily pleasure. As he demands "milk," or "candy" or "water," the word-names are repeated for him. These word-names are not put into sentences; they are not spoken with questioning inflection; they are not requested of the learner; they are merely repeated many times over as the child requests and receives the object of his desires. By limiting the number of objects named for the learner to the few satisfying objects that are commonly received every day and perhaps many times a day, stimulation is given in a very restricted area. The associations set up by this very simple Pavlovian approach are frequently sufficient to establish the word-name as a substitute for the object. Once this has been done successfully, it has been the author's experience with normal children that language develops rather rapidly with simple word-illustrations.

Concentration on a Few Words.—Following somewhat the same technique with the aphasic adult, it has been found most successful to limit the number of word-names to a relatively small list. The names most easily learned are representative of objects that give the patient the greatest amount of pleasure. For one patient, learning the name "radio" and the name "pencil" was enough to establish the naming process, and other names were added with comparative ease. The method used to establish the two names mentioned was to (a) indicate the article by pointing to it; (b) repeat the name several times; (c) turn the radio on and listen to something for a moment with the patient; (d) repeat a series of other names and have the patient select the word "radio" from the others (the manner of this selection was usually her reaching over to the radio when the word-name was enunciated); (e) show the word "radio" printed on a card in letters four inches high (the patient had an alexia and could not read); (f) have the patient trace the printed word as the name was repeated; (g) encourage the patient for every little effort made in attempting to enunciate the word-name; and (h) point to the radio upon entering the room and indicate that the patient should name it. These and countless other little suggestive clews were used to elicit the name. The word-finding game was played at every session just as the contact started. As other procedures were used for different attacks on the generalized problem, the word "radio" was introduced whenever possible. For instance, in writing training for agraphia, the word "radio" was traced many times, and each tracing was accompanied by the therapist's repetition of the word-name. Selection of objects in the room for training in visual form recognition always included the radio. Nurses and attendants were instructed to use the word whenever it was meaningfully possible. With all of this effort directed toward this one word-name (plus a series of three other common objects), the patient first enunciated the word some three months after training was started. At about the same time the word "book" was produced, as was "pencil." Following the production of these words, other words returned rapidly, and within a period of two weeks the patient could name almost any common object within her training area. This extended to less commonly seen objects in a short time, until the naming process was almost complete at the end of the fifth month.

General Principles of Therapy.—This long illustration is used to indicate many of the principles that seem to be operating in the reeducation process. First, use every possible clue and cue. Second, be patient and accepting of every effort. Third, do not stay too long in any one session on the word-finding effort. Fourth, use every person that comes in contact with the patient to assist in the naming process. Fifth, do not urge the use of names on the part of the patient, teach by example. Sixth, imitation of the therapist's use of a name does not appear to be helpful, therefore the therapist should discourage parrot-like repetition. Seventh, give the patient every opportunity to use the name before applying the word. Eighth, stay at the word level if possible; building words by similar phonetic endings is a lengthy process that is rarely helpful in establishing the recall necessary for speech.

Patience is the greatest single virtue of the aphasia therapist, and in no other area is it more necessary than in that of resolving the anomia problem.

Dysarthria

Another defect in speech that is common to all types of aphasia patients is the inability to produce repetitive muscular movements of articulation in a smooth and rhythmical fashion. When this is present without peripheral paralysis or injury, the cause is said to be cortical and due to a damaged motor process in the cortex. It is a commonly seen counterpart of aphasia, although it is not infrequently seen when the usual aphasic manifestations are absent. The consequences of the disability are seen in the articulatory production of speech. On the test form discussed in Chapter 8, the patient is asked to repeat after the examiner such words as "cross," "triangle," "seven," "Massachusetts," and "Methodist Episcopal." These words are used because of the ascending degree of difficulty presented in their articulation. Where the first three will elicit articulatory difficulty only in the most dysarthric patient, the last two and especially the last item will elicit the problem in a great majority of patients. Common manifestations on the word-pair "Methodist Episcopal" are such attempts as "medosis epitopul," "mesosis epitopul," and "mesosis episopil." The tongue-movements are found to be sluggish, confused, and sometimes totally absent.

Differentiating Facial Paralysis from Cortical Disorder.—It is often necessary to differentiate between the common dysarthria found in the paralyzed patient and the cortical type of the disorder, for many aphasic patients show a facial paralysis which may affect the articulatory musculature, especially the tongue and lips. The most common differentiating sign is the production of vowels, especially in terms of vowel length. The facially paralyzed patient is inclined to drawl his words and to articulate in sound or syllable groups, while the central dysarthrias appear in the failure to enunciate consonant sounds. Both types show final elisions and frequently paraphasic reversals of sounds or what appear to be substitutions of sounds. Usually the latter are not true substitutions but are sounds made by tongue-movements which are just not rapid enough to keep up with the articulatory effort. Thus, medial consonant combinations will be reduced to single consonants, while consonants will be eliminated or elided to prepare the muscles for the following word.

Training Procedures.—Direct training for rapidity of muscular movements is sometimes helpful. Repetition of such syllables as *la* or *ta;* upward, downward, and sidewise movements of the tongue are sometimes helpful. Recognition of errors made by use of recordings of speech attempts, explanation and discussion of the problem until the patient can conceive of his own problem, and other simple speech techniques have been used with some success. By and large, however, recovery from dysarthria that is central in origin usually accompanies aphasia recovery without any individual effort or with little more than simple suggestion at the later stages of training.

In the present context it is proposed that the area of dysarthria is one of the few places where phonetic training techniques may be of some value. In the main, however, accuracy in enunciation has been considered as the least of the problems confronting the aphasic adult. The author has never insisted upon correctness in articulation as an early goal for the patient. Rather it is felt that the ability to express one's self in free and easy speech and the use of all of the communicating forms of language are the important areas for the therapist to consider. Accuracy of enunciation is a comparatively easy, although specialized, area which can be treated separately if necessary, after the patient has learned to function on an adult level in terms of ability to use speech and language. For this reason the part that training for dysarthria takes in the present proposed training program is minimized and dealt with only during the later stages of training.

Paraphasia

The residual speech of many aphasic patients, as well as the recovered speech both during and after therapy, often shows grammatical lapses and confused enunciation. These errors of syntax and articulatory omissions or confusions are called *paraphasic disturbances*. Analysis of the patient's speech will show that the errors are due to sound, syllable, and even whole-word substitutions, reversals, or omissions. Paraphasia is found in all of the categories of aphasia. Two types can be described. While they are most often seen in particular aphasic groups, they may appear interchangeably in the same patient and therefore should not be considered pathognomonic. The following operational definitions should prove useful.

Paraphasia.—A generic term, it describes all types of apparent errors of syntax or grammatical form found in the speech or writing of aphasic patients.

Agrammatism.—This is the paraphasic disorder most frequently seen in the expressive aphasias. The specific disorder of grammar is one in which all or most of the "grammatical" words of the language are omitted. The speech is often called "telegram-style" or "telegraphic speech" because of its similarity to the style used in writing telegrams where all nonuseful words are eliminated. When such words as "the," "on," "a," "to," etc., are present, they are often used incorrectly. (For examples see text below.)

Paragrammatism.—This paraphasic disorder is most often seen in the receptive aphasias. The form this disturbance takes is that of substitution, reversal, or omission of sounds or syllables within a word or reversal of words within a sentence. The sound reversals, substitutions, or omissions are most often within a particular word. The syllable substitutions, reversals, or omissions most often affect the suffixes and prefixes. When whole words are affected, there may be a relation between the word used and its correct form in meaning, category, or phoneme. This relationship, however, is commonly not seen. When paragrammatism is present to a marked degree, the speech may be largely unintelligible. (For examples see text below.)

Examples of Paragrammatism.—The first of these language problems is noted most often as a defect common to the receptive aphasic patient. Examples from patient's histories may serve to simplify the type of disorder and to some degree indicate the therapy which has been most useful. A recent patient when shown a picture of a key and asked to explain its function after naming it, responded, "Open. You open out when you want to come in there, see?" He demonstrated the act and then said, "Let's see—kitten. You mean how near can I get it. Let's see—kitten. It starts with a kit—kidder." That is a rather typical receptive aphasic patient's response pattern. The first response was related to the function of a key in a door. The attempt to secure the actual name was paraphasic— the use of "kitten," "kit," and "kidder" was phonetically related to the stimulus "key" through the initial k sound. The inability to

recognize the error of the attempt was an indication of the receptive
nature of the response, a lack of self-criticism of verbal language.

Another patient showed a typical paragrammatic type of error
in her reversal of the first sound in a pair of words. The sentence
form "pencil write" was produced as "wencil pites." The same patient tended to reverse whole syllables by saying, "He shouting the
warned" instead of "He shouted the warning." At times these substitutions and confusions result in such garbled speech efforts that
most speech attempts seem like almost pure jargon speech. So prev-
alent was this in some of the earliest descriptions of speech seen by
Jackson that he predicated a complete category of language disturbance which he called "jargon aphasia." [11]

Examples of Agrammatism.—Examples of the agrammatism
common to the expressive aphasic patient show the expected shorten-
ing of sentence form, the tendency to reverse words in sentences, and
the use of the wrong words for the context. One patient recovered
speech in general rather rapidly but could not obtain a real understanding of grammatical form. Sentences were used both in speech
and in writing that demonstrated her difficulty. The articles "a" and
"the" were used at times, but as frequently incorrectly as correctly.
In commenting on the family car and her afternoon ride she would
say "We drive a car," "A car downtown," "I and she ride car," and
"A hill is far away." The verb "to be" was very confusing to her,
and only after many hours of work did it begin to be used meaningfully. An example of her use of the verb would be "The phonograph
is the record" or "The man is a coat." At times she would reverse
the word order and the same sentences would be written "A record
is a phonograph" or "A coat is a man." Prepositions, articles, and
conjunctions were difficult grammatical forms for her to conquer.
For many months sentences were used eliminating all but the noun
or pronoun, the verb, and possibly an object. Prepositional phrases,
the correct use of the article or the conjunction, and the need for a
full grammatical sentence were exceedingly difficult concepts.

Still another example of agrammatism is commonly seen, the
tendency to omit sounds. One patient whose articulation in terms
of his ability to produce all of the sounds of the language was exceedingly good would substitute consonants in the middle of a word.
The word "sky" would be pronounced as "sty" or "spy." The sentence "The sky is blue" would be pronounced as "The sty is bool,"

---

[11] J. H. Jackson, "Hughlings Jackson on Aphasia," edited by H. Head, *Brain*,
XXXVIII (1915), 8–29.

while "The stars are shining" was spoken as "The skars are sined." An extension of this type of speech is barely intelligible and in some instances wholly unintelligible.

Therapy for Word Disorders.—While it has been stated that these specific language and syntactical problems are most likely to appear in one form or another of the aphasia seen in adults, they are rarely exclusive and cannot be considered as completely pathognomonic of type or classification. In general it must be remembered that these disorders are tenacious and difficult to overcome. Therapy has usually been direct, through phonetic training for the reversals or confusions within the word. Phonetic training in this instance is directed not at articulation but at auditory discrimination and recognition of error. Some success can be obtained by writing the speech used for later analysis by the patient. Through their own concentration on the manner in which their speech attempts are heard and some care in speaking, many patients are able to obviate the greater part of their misuse of sounds within words. For the syntactical errors, training in grammar and in grammatical form is sometimes useful, especially in those patients with a good pretraumatic grounding in academic pursuits. One previous school-teacher was able to master syntax through the application of common grammatical rules. Ordinarily, however, the patient's reaction to grammatical rules is not salutary. Resolution of the difficulty comes, when it comes at all, during the later stages of training, when errors can be perceived and corrected directly in the speech attempts. The use of recorded speech, with the patient listening to his own speech attempts, may also prove useful on some occasions. By and large direct attempts to correct or to train patients showing these disorders are difficult and not too productive.

Expressive-Receptive and Global Aphasia

To complete our overview of therapy for different types of aphasic patients, it remains to discuss briefly two more groups of patients, the mixed expressive-receptive and the global aphasic. The first of these is the type of patient who shows a severe aphasic disturbance in the areas of both reception and expression, with little to choose between them in regard to the predominance of symptoms.

Expressive-Receptive Aphasics.—These patients show such a widespread disorder that the therapist, despite his planned intentions, must adjust his goals to very near language possibilities rather than to the far-off stages of eventual recovery. For these patients it has been found most useful to attempt to determine at the outset a single area of language that is useful to the patient. If he responds best to visual clues, the therapist should follow that avenue in the early stages of training. For instance, a patient showing mixed aphasia had retained as his one least affected receptive area the ability to follow simple instructions when presented to him visually through the medium of visual forms and signs. Totally alexic and unable to gain any understanding from verbal directions, he could recognize visual forms such as the meaning of directional arrows, and fortunately he did not have a body agnosia. Training was instituted using gross geometrical forms from a design representing in gross outline the figure of a person, with a circle for the head, a rectangle for the body, two large triangles for the legs, and two small ones for the arms. Features were added by using small squares for eyes, an elongated rectangle for the mouth, a small triangle for the nose, and two small circles for ears. These various parts of the figure were related to the parts of his body, and names were attached to them visually by rote-learning and repetition. The use of each part was shown by acting out the function of the parts without verbal language first; thus the eyes were shown to be visual organs, the nose for smelling, etc. The patient was encouraged to cut out such a figure in paper and later in wood. These self-constructed figures were made to represent people in the environment. As recognition proceeded from the constructed figures, names for each part were added through visual and oral presentation. From this inauspicious starting point, reading was started, and oral reproduction of visually presented words was made an immediate goal. Language in general was introduced only after reading and verbal reception were achieved at a useful stage.

The patient showing a mixed type of aphasia should be treated in much the same manner as the one showing a predominantly expressive or predominantly receptive aphasia as soon as a proper avenue of relation and understanding has been achieved.

Therapy for the Global Aphasic.—A similar approach is necessary for the global-aphasic patient. Here the patient exhibits almost a complete lack of relation with the environment. It is usually impossible to determine the severity of any individual phase of his problem. The differentiating characteristic between these patients and the severe mixed aphasic patient is only one of degree. Probably the one major diagnostic sign is the presence of some observable retained language function in the mixed expressive-receptive type. The global patient may well possess a series of automatic verbalizations or some rather extensive "jargon" language but shows little if any useful language retention.

The usual course of treatment with these patients is to attempt to stimulate them in constantly changing ways. One patient responded rather well to brightly colored objects but apparently was unable to comprehend or to respond to material despite his interest. However, a continuous use of colored material found him reacting in a typical infantile fashion. He would attempt to follow verbal directions with the material but usually could do nothing but imitate a selection rather than follow the direction. After recognizing the additional stimulation that came from using multicolored material, however, the therapist ingeniously varied the material until it was found that the patient had developed a game of his own when the material was left with him. The squares, circles, oblongs, and diamonds of bright wood, such as the Vigotsky blocks or the Kohs blocks, which were left with the patient in an unassorted mass each day were always sorted into a rather good combination series on the therapist's return the following day. Using the sorting principle developed by the patient, which usually was one based upon color rather than size or depth, the therapist perseverated with color-naming exercises each day. After a considerable period the patient was found attempting to imitate the names given the primary colors by the therapist. While his attempts were not accurate, they were distinctly symbolic representations. As time and spontaneous physical recovery went on, it was found that within the patient's limited articulatory skill he could name the colors red and blue with some consistency and the colors yellow and white occasionally. Other material was introduced in the first two colors named, and a transfer was made from the blocks to pictures of more meaningful material. Animals of different shape, but always in red or blue, were shown, and by association the names for the animals were attached. Thus the patient learned to recognize and to say "red horse" and "blue cat." It was a direct step forward when colors were discontinued and the names "horse" and "cat" were retained. From animals in pictures the patient was able to master other named objects like "boy," "saddle," "dog," etc., all appearing with the original animals. Language training was then made more general, and the global characteristics seemed to disappear as the patient gained a rapid recognition and a slower verbal ability. The patient was then treated as a typical expressive aphasic adult.

The major point to be seen in these mixed expressive-receptive and global aphasic patients is that at the onset of training there must be found some avenue of entry into the patient's consciousness, some avenue of sufficient interest to the patient that he will continue to respond through the lengthy and rather monotonous early stages. Once a pathway is discovered and some progress is made, however, it is often found that the problem rather quickly resolves itself into either a typical expressive or a receptive language problem which can be treated in the same fashion as other problems of that type.

Summary of Aphasia Therapy

The suggestions and illustrations given in the last two chapters show the double significance of all language training for aphasic adults. The therapist must recognize at all times that, while he attacks a particular disability in communication skill, he is at the same time dealing psychotherapeutically with a readjusting personality. Just as it is impossible to devise therapeusis that affects only one of the facets of the total problem, so is it impossible to deal with and to treat only the communication problem. Communication can only exist as a need within the need-structure of an individual. His interpersonal relations and his attitudes toward self and toward the world he lives in are constantly in flux and readjusting. Recovery from aphasia requires growth toward stability, toward acceptance of self, toward a continuing opportunity for self-expression. Every contact between therapist and patient is a therapeutic one, and the therapist must always be alert to every opportunity to assist the patient in whichever direction he may turn.

Successful reduction of aphasic language disturbances is dependent upon a multitude of factors, among which are early diagnosis and referral; careful analysis of the retained and disturbed language functions; proper evaluation of the nonlanguage behavior characteristics; insight into the basic personality of the patient; persistence and patience on the part of the therapist; and cooperation of all of the possible human elements in the patient's immediate environment. The aphasia therapist must be psychologist, speech pathologist, and educator. He must look for and use the services of the family, friends, physicians, neurologists, electroencephalographers, physiotherapists, and occupational therapists. Most important of all, he must be able to coordinate all of the assistance he receives for the ultimate growth of the patient. Despite the awesome nature of the above admonition, the basic task must be recognized as one in which the therapist serves essentially to assist nature in its readjustment to an incomplete cortex as the individual strives to recapture his innate language and adjustmental abilities. All recovery, the author feels, is dependent upon retained structure and cortical potential—within the limitations of the patient's personality percepts. Therapy to be ultimately and maximally effective must be supportive of the individual's striving toward stability—the goal of all people at all times.

Chapter 14

ILLUSTRATIVE CASE MATERIAL

Some of the theoretical concepts concerning aphasia therapy as well as the application of some of the therapeutic techniques can best be illustrated through a review of case histories. Aphasia patients are to be found in many different circumstances, and consequently two widely different approaches will be shown. The first case from the writer's files is that of a head-wounded soldier seen in the Aphasia Center described earlier. It demonstrates the therapeusis possible in a total-push, inpatient environment. The second case is one seen since the recent war. It exemplifies the out-patient, in-the-home therapeutic approach. In any instance it should be recalled as the author's opinion that all therapy for aphasia must be on an individual level. It should be based upon the expressed and observed needs of the patient and not on any predetermined academic goal-level established by the therapist. Generalizations in therapy can only concern approaches to specific portions of the presenting problem. Often the approach used will depend upon such factors as the availability of the patient to the therapist; the proximity and availability of other resources such as physiotherapy, occupational therapy, and the like; the living space occupied by the patient; and, unfortunately, such extraneous factors as the economic condition of the patient. No easy solution to these facets of the problem of aphasia therapy are immediately apparent. They may find eventual resolution, it is believed, through extension of aphasia therapy to increasing numbers of patients and the consequent recognition by society of the need for such therapeusis.

The immediately preceding chapters on direct language therapy have shown some of the techniques found useful by the author in specific instances of demonstrable apraxias and agnosias. It is hoped that the implication of a fractionated and specific therapy has not been drawn from this presentation. Actually, it is strongly held by the present writer that therapy should be generalized to the whole patient in every possible way, rather than made specific to his particular disability. The person, the whole person, and not the deficiencies must be treated. In another sense, too, should therapy be

249

generalized. Multiple-sense stimuli should be utilized rather than isolated direct appeals to one medium. The possibility of obtaining motivation and direct learning through minimal clues in even the most evidently disturbed function should not be overlooked. The pathways to recovery for aphasia are not yet so clearly established that any media leading to comprehension or expression of language or self should not be tried.

A Case of Expressive Aphasia

The patient was a twenty-four-year-old single male, wounded six months previously. His referral diagnosis was "Encephalopathy, posttraumatic due to penetrating gunshot wound in the left frontoparietal region which produced a complete right hemiplegia, hemianesthesia, and aphasia." The accompanying record showed that the patient on the day of his injury was "stuporous and out of contact." On that day his wound was "debrided and bony fragments and macerated brain tissue were flushed out." Three weeks later, the record said, "the wound was explored and found to contain cloudy fluids."

On admission to the treatment hospital it was noted that "the hemiplegia had improved slightly, especially in the lower extremity. The upper extremity remained almost completely paralyzed. Examination reveals a large pulsating defect 5 × 8 cms. in the left frontoparietal region, a continuous tinnitus in both ears, a right homonymous hemianopsia, hemihypesthesia, and aphasia." The patient was referred to the Aphasia Center for evaluation and therapy if indicated.

On the first visit to the Center the patient was studied by a receiving psychologist who administered a screening test for organic impairment. The following results were obtained:

A. Vocabulary—average adult level (measurement through multiple choice and gesture, since no spoken language was available to patient)

B. Visual recall—poor

C. Attention and concentration—poor (below testable levels)

D. Visual object recall—poor (2 of 10 objects recalled)

E. Personal memory—(1) Immediate—very poor

(2) Recent—fair (2 of 6 items showed accurate recall)

(3) Old—good with only slight inaccuracies

F. Writing—prints name only with left hand (hemiplegic)

G. Reading—poor (below any standard test level; no recall)

H. Visual perception—satisfactory within limits of hemianopsia

I. Visual abstraction ability—good

Impression: Impairment generalized, especially in spheres of productive speech, kinesthesias, attention and concentration, personal memory, reading, and writing; comprehension good.

Following sessions were taken up with a language examination. An aphasia screening test was administered with the following results:

A. Agnosias—(1) Visual word agnosia—moderate
             (2) Audio-visuo-kinetic agnosia—moderate
             (3) Body agnosia—moderate
B. Apraxias—(1) Verbal apraxia—severe
             (2) Number apraxia—severe
             (3) Calculation apraxia—severe
             (4) Construction apraxia—moderate
             (5) Ideokinetic apraxia—moderate
C. Anomia—severe
D. Dysarthria—not testable
E. Paraphasia—not testable

Impression: Expressive aphasia—severe, with almost generalized complete loss in every motor act of language with the exception of agraphia and general (nonverbal) apraxia. Writing difficult because of hemiplegia. Receptive signs present, but moderate in nature, especially seen in areas of reading, following more than simple instruction and in body relationships. Referral for language therapy was recommended.

A review of the available army records showed that the patient had a pretraumatic Army General Classification Test score of Class III—106; that he had completed ten grades of school in a rural community in California; and that his prearmy occupation had been that of a farmhand and general laborer.

A staff conference decided that therapy should begin immediately, with the initial emphasis placed upon verbal expression at the single-word-naming level, with simultaneous work in reading and writing. Occupational therapy and physiotherapy were delayed at the request of the neurologist because of impending neurosurgery.

After two weeks in the Center and the establishment of beginning rapport with the members of the staff, the initial stage of intelligence and achievement testing was undertaken with the following results:[1]

A. Intelligence testing (Wechsler-Bellevue adult intelligence scale)
    Totals obtained—Verbal score—70
                      Performance score—92
                      Full scale—79

The test scatter obtained showed the following pattern:

Verbal Tests	(Weighted Scores)	Performance Tests	(Weighted Scores)
Information	10	Picture arrangement	10
Comprehension	5	Picture completion	9
Digits	4	Block design	8
Arithmetic	0	Object assembly	10
Similarities	4	Digit symbol	8
Total	23	Total	45
(Vocabulary	9)		

---

[1] The test scores given are based upon the examiner's estimate in many instances since the questions asked often called for direct oral response. The scores are consequently considered as subjective approximations rather than as direct objective statements of the patient's ability.

B. Educational achievement testing (progressive achievement test)

Reading   Grade 1
Writing   Grade 1
Spelling   Grade 1.5
Mathematics Grade 2

C. Speech performance (based on rating scale, page 53)
Level 1 (scale runs from 1 to 5, where 5 is normal speech)

During the ensuing two months therapy was given on an individual basis. Visual stimulation by pictures and objects with minimal phonetic clues was used in the direct verbal work. A picture or object selected by the patient would be placed in front of him, the name would be spoken and printed on the blackboard, and the use of the object would be described through sign, motion, and gesture. The patient would be asked to respond in any way possible, either by naming the object if he could, or by printing the name as he attempted to sound it, or by indicating its use. His general euphoria and almost complete lack of emotional frustration at failure made it possible to extend the stimulus periods to fairly long forty- and fifty-minute periods. Writing was started by the use of Gardner's left-handed writing manual. Practice with the basic circles and lines was discontinued after the first session because of the evident lack of motivation. Script writing was seen to be extremely difficult and nonproductive; consequently the patient was permitted to print. The same words presented in the verbal therapy were used as practice for writing. In reading it was noted that only nouns and direct-action verbs could be comprehended. Reading material was constructed by the therapist, using the stimulus words of the verbal therapy. During these two months a steady and encouraging progress was noted in language usage of the verbal type. No increase in reading ability was observed. Writing remained at the printing level.

Following a two-week break for neurosurgery the patient returned to therapy. It was noted that the euphoria had decreased, but that no real anxiety was evidenced. The patient appeared to be more alert and better able to concentrate. Physiotherapy and occupational therapy were begun. Both approaches seemed to stimulate the patient. A slight regression was noted in his oral speech attempts during the first postoperative week. This loss was seen to be temporary, however, since the patient was soon able to respond at his previous level.

Sentence-completion exercises were used in all three spheres of language training. This work was correlated with the occupational therapy program. For example, the patient evidenced considerable interest in weaving and in leather-plaiting, and consequently sentences constructed for the patient's completion were on the following order: "We weave with ———"; "The weaving machine is called a ———"; "The color of the wool is ———"; "We can make a ——— on the loom"; "Belts are made of ———"; "The leather comes in ———." The missing words were demonstrated in oral and visual form, and similar words were written and supplied orally. Multiple-choice selection was necessary at first but later could be discontinued as the patient's ability to name objects spontaneously was seen to improve.

By the end of the next month it was noted that verbs and nouns could be combined into short sentences in both speech and writing. Script instead of printing was taught, and only in reading was a lack of progress noted. The patient remained cooperative and conscientious. Small-group therapy in spelling was added to the therapeusis. A list of spelling words attempted at this time included the following: hen, cow, pen, horse, man, ball, farm, mother, hello, walk, talk. The attempt was made to relate the spelling to the patient's previous experience and interest. At first only the first three words of the list could be spelled with accuracy. Phonetic training was given in the group, and spelling was made a part of daily therapy. It was found that words used in other areas of training were more easily spelled and more meaningful to the patient; consequently such words as "loom," "leather," "wool," etc., were used and it was seen that motivation increased and spelling ability seemed to move ahead rapidly.

Two months after the operation noted above, the patient was observed in a *grand mal* Jacksonian-type seizure. No aura was evidenced. The patient was unconscious for approximately fifteen minutes. Fatigue seemed to be the only immediate after-effect. Therapy was continued on the following day without further interruption. This was the first seizure seen at the Center. With the patient's permission it was discussed in a group with eight other patients. The likelihood of seizures, the effect of having them, the purposes of medication, and the need for continuing medication were all brought up. (From this time on, these eight patients formed a group which discussed common problems of brain-injured patients three times each week. These particular men were selected for this first group largely because of the indications that they were the most outgoing of the patient population and evidenced signs of real leadership. Later they became the nucleus of several other groups that were formed. Eventually every patient in the Center was included. The formation of these small groups for discussion seemed to serve as excellent motivation for the over-all therapy.)

With the success obtained in small-group therapy, as in spelling, all training for this patient was changed to the group approach with the exception of reading. In this area one hour of individual training was given each day. Writing, verbal expression, and spelling were given in different-sized groups. Verbal expression as a direct approach was supplemented by the conversational method used in the discussion group. The direct language training for development of voluntary speech was approached through the two-patient group method. This patient and one other at approximately the same level of language met together with the therapist. After a short beginning devoted to review of previous constructs such as naming, verb-usage, and sentence completion, the two would compete against each other in conversational attempts. For example, a short sentence would be started by the therapist and completed by the first patient able to produce the desired or a desirable complete sentence. Words would be written on the board and each patient would attempt to find a synonym or antonym that he could say. Difficult words were started by the therapist and completed by the patients. Throughout a friendly spirit of competition was maintained with a daily record of success kept. The only reward used was therapist approval and patient recognition of success.

It was found that the patient could accomplish more at this time in both speech and writing if the two were used simultaneously. In consequence, writing the desired word or sentence before speaking it was encouraged. Since the patient evidenced an interest in numbers at this time, a beginning approach to number usage was instituted. The patient's partner in verbal expression followed this patient's interest, and the two-patient approach was used from the onset in this area.

Reading remained the most difficult problem. Some improvement was noted, however, in this area as soon as the patient's verbal expression improved to the short-sentence stage. To maintain motivation, since this patient did so well in group activity, he was paired with another patient for reading. This proved to be very salutory. Both patients showed an immediate improvement. They selected their own material from the Center library and worked on comprehension by writing difficult words down, by breaking them into syllables, by sounding, and by flash card or tachistoscopic exposures. By the end of two months of paired reading work, this area had improved to the level of the patient's other language functions.

Writing had advanced to the personal-letter stage. The patient was encouraged to compose letters to his family, his friends in other wards, and his friends in other parts of the army and at home. While the patient indicated that letter-writing had never been one of his strong points before his injury, he now wanted to write to everyone he knew. His first letters were rarely two sentences long. While he wanted to write, he could never find anything to say except short declarative statements about his speech, his health, and his limitation of movement. He was encouraged to expand his ideas in writing, to describe the training and his daily activities, and later to express his thoughts and feelings. Letter-writing remained a favorite form of writing training for this patient. (This was in direct opposition to most of the patients at the Center, who rarely attempted to send out any of the letters they composed in the therapeutic sessions.)

After eight months of therapy, a re-evaluation of the patient's problem was made. Social service had completed a survey of the patient's background and home environment. While the background was not directly contributory, it gave the therapists some immediate insights that could not be obtained from the patient. An abstract of the social history showed:

"Patient was the second of two brothers. He was born on a farm in South Dakota and moved to California when quite young. His closest family relationship was with his mother, who was found to be a warm, affectionate woman, a good housekeeper, and the major stabilizing force in the home. The father was a good provider, kind-hearted and close to both of his sons.

"The patient had a 'normal' childhood. He had had the usual childhood diseases, but no serious illnesses. He was always gregarious and exceptionally well liked by his peers. He was a leader in his high school, but always was described as being modest and somewhat passive and retiring when placed in positions of responsibility. He succeeded at everything he attempted but never wanted or sought external recognition. After finishing two years of high school he thought that he had had enough and went to work on a farm. His present plans are, first, to continue with his language training as long as he continues to progress. Then to return home to his family where there is an opportunity to work in a store run by his brother.

"The family seems extraordinarily understanding of the patient's condition and with some orientation should be able to provide the type of home that would be very good for the patient."

The re-evaluation in language showed generalized improvement. The recovery process seemed to have good momentum. In verbal expression there was an improving ability to use language freely. Sentences were commonly used. Writing had become free and easy, and the patient could write almost everything he could say. Reading had improved to the point where fourth-grade material (or material of a nonacademic nature judged to be about at the level of a ten-year-old) could be read with fair comprehension and retention. Mathematics and use of numbers was still noted at the beginning level. Attention and concentration were still affected. In occupational therapy great strides had been made. Physiotherapy reported that the patient's hemiplegia had been reduced in the lower extremity to the point where walking was easy, although a foot-drop was still present and a brace was still necessary. The staff conference decided to continue the patient in therapy. Emphasis, it was decided, should be placed on the higher intellectual processes, mainly through the pathway of group discussion and competitive language therapy. All phases of training should be continued and a beginning made toward off-the-ward and out-of-the-hospital socialization.

Therapy was continued along the lines indicated. Increased motivation was seen in the socialization efforts. The patient made biweekly trips into the near-by city, either in company with other aphasic patients or alone. He was encouraged to talk to people, to shop in various stores, to seek out a local friend, and to engage strangers in conversation. Most of these tasks he accomplished well as time went on. He became a leader in his own discussion group. As the second president of a social club formed by the patients in the Aphasia Center, he found increased opportunity to use language at a high plane. Through card-playing he began to show an increased familiarity with numbers and their usages. He continued to show some spelling difficulty, and a separate hour a day was devoted to this subject. Since phonetics seemed to be the one useful approach for this patient, it was stressed. He constructed with the aid of the occupational therapist a workbook of his own manufacture in which he kept a daily record of each phoneme as he studied it. Because of his wide interest in affairs of the day, reading took the form of daily newspaper study. He displayed a greater interest in this stimulus than in book-reading. In mathematics the patient's expressed interest in returning to a merchant's role after hospital discharge was utilized. He showed a progression through fractions and decimals after this device was instituted.

At the end of eighteen months of intensive training a complete analysis of his ability was made with the following results:

A. Intelligence testing (Wechsler-Bellevue adult intelligence scale)

Verbal score	102	
Performance score	104	
Full scale	109	(Classification: Average adult)

The individual weighted scores showed the following distribution:

Information	13	Picture arrangement	14
Comprehension	15	Picture completion	12
Digits	4	Block design	10
Arithmetic	10	Object assembly	10
Similarities	14	Digit symbol	7
Total	56	Total	53
Vocabulary	16		

B. Language testing (aphasia test)

Verbal apraxia—mild
Calculation apraxia—mild
Anomia—mild
Alexia—mild

C. Educational achievement (progressive achievement test)

Reading	9th grade level
Writing	11th grade level
Spelling	10th grade level
Mathematics	10th grade level

D. Speech performance (rating scale, page 53)
Level 4 (on scale from 1 to 5, where 5 is normal speech)

The improvement shown by the patient in every area indicated to the staff of the Center that successful rehabilitation for this patient could be achieved. It was felt that it was time that he moved from the somewhat overprotective and sheltered existence of a hospital to his home. Plans were made for an over-all discussion with the parents preparing them for the return of the patient. It was recommended to the medical authorities that this patient had received maximum benefit of hospitalization; that his impairment was only minimal; that he was competent to handle his own affairs; and that he had a residual aphasia which might improve to some extent, but probably would always be somewhat debilitating. A continuance of physiotherapy and a vocational plan were discussed with the patient prior to his discharge.

Follow-up: Since the patient's discharge from the hospital and the Aphasia Center, he has been in contact with the writer many times. He has made an excellent social and vocational adjustment. He is occupied in running a general store, keeps his own accounts, has a part ownership of a farm, and spends part of his time assisting them. The right arm and hand are still markedly paralyzed; the leg, however, is improved, and locomotion is no great problem. Considerable speech improvement is noted in free verbal expression. The academic subject material, however, remains at approximately the level that it was on discharge from the hospital. Letters from the patient indicate a remaining difficulty in spelling and a tendency to substitute words. Writing intelligibility is good, but the rate of writing is slow. The patient's attitude and control of affect remain good; he is well liked in his community and seems to be as rehabilitated as an individual can be within the confines of his physical limitations.

A Case of Expressive-Receptive Aphasia

The patient was a fifty-nine-year-old married mother of one child. The referral diagnosis was "Cerebrovascular accident with resultant right hemiplegia and aphasia." The brain injury had occurred ten months prior to referral. The patient was not ambulatory.

The pretraumatic history was given by the patient's husband. It was noted that the patient had been a school-teacher for many years. She was a university graduate and had specialized in early elementary education. She had written many books for children and for teachers at the level of beginning reading. She had founded schools for progressive educational techniques at the beginning level of education. She had always been very forthright in her attitudes toward liberal movements both in education and in social thought. While no self-seeker for glory or self-recognition, she had led many movements for teachers' rights and for equality of opportunity. She had been noted for her intense interests, her high intellectual ability, and her consistent pleasantness, coupled with her unshaking opposition to anything that impeded social change and improvement.

Avocationally, it was noted that she liked classical music, classical art, travel, and literary pursuits. Other forms of music, art, and literature were disliked almost as much as the former were appreciated. While home-making and the multitude of activities that preoccupy the home-maker were engaged in, they were never the major interest of her life. She had many friends of long standing in the higher intellectual social groups of the city.

Therapy was planned for on a five-times-a-week basis. This plan was followed for eighteen months. Since the response patterns of the patient were so limited and the evident aphasia was so widespread, formal examination of language was dispensed with and direct therapy was instituted immediately.

The first examination revealed a pleasant, smiling, bedridden woman who could comprehend almost nothing that was said to her directly. She indicated her immediate wants to her nurse by pointing or by gestures which were usually understood after a series of repetitions. She was euphoric most of the time; had a comparatively short attention-span; tried to cooperate with the examiner, but became easily frustrated and showed some emotional withdrawal after a few attempts to respond ended in failure. She evidenced some understanding of spoken words when they were not direct requests made to her that required response. For example, when the examiner commented to the nurse that it was quite warm in the room, the patient shook her head several times. As the nurse, who had not been observing the patient's reactions at that moment, went to open the window, the head-shaking gesture was repeated. When the nurse then put the window down, the patient immediately responded by smiling and nodding her head. She could respond to simple direct suggestions such as "Look at the window" and "Turn your head to the wall." She could respond to only one of a pair of such requests, however. When asked to "Look at the radio and then at the window," she responded by looking at the radio, but was confused when attempting the second request. She made no vocal attempts other than repetition of the vowel *i*. She used this sound repetitively many times. When she wanted to attract the nurse's attention, she would repeat the vowel several times. She did not inflect the sound as though substituting it for conversation or for verbal communication. No automatic phrases were used. She was noted as being hemiplegic, even needing some help in turning over in bed. Her health was reported as good; her blood pressure normal; her food intake low, but sufficient. She was under medication (phenobarbital, grains 1, three times a day).

The early sessions were taken up with short periods of familiarization with the therapist. The first stage of training began during the second week. The therapist would indicate objects in the room and name them. The patient would attempt to respond by imitation without success. Such objects as glass, water, bed, pencil, and clock were indicated and named. Each time that a series of names was used and the objects indicated, they would be gone over again without being named. Thus, the pencil would be shown and named, the patient attempting to say the word in imitation. Usually, no vocalization was achieved other than *i*. At the same time it was noted that if the examiner indicated the pencil and called it improperly, the patient would shake her head sidewise, then when the correct name was used, she would respond by saying *i* and nodding her head up and down. The pencil would then be shown but not named. The writing act would be demonstrated and the word "pencil" would be written on a blackboard or a large piece of white paper. The pencil would be placed in the patient's hand (the left hand) and the paper placed so she could attempt to write with it. During all of these later examples the word "pencil" would be repeated several times with each act. This process of continuous naming was explained to the nurse and to the husband. Each time the opportunity arose during the day, whenever water was desired, for example, or the patient wished the bed raised or lowered, or the time of day was mentioned, the appropriate naming word was to be repeated several times. The patient was not to be asked to repeat the word, and questioning inflection was not to be used as the word was repeated by others.

After some two months of this naming therapy, the patient attempted her first complete word. On pointing to the glass of water next to her bed she said "water." This was shortly followed by a series of other word attempts. Within two weeks the patient could add new words almost as soon as they were given to her but could not initiate any of them, with the exception of a short series which had been used repeatedly throughout the therapeusis until that time. Therapeutic sessions were constructed of word-naming periods accompanied by writing and beginning reading of the same words. Each session would begin with a review of the names for the common objects in the room. Then new word-names would be added for additional objects. New words were added successfully only when the object could be visualized. Attempts to secure successful naming of objects that could not be seen was completely futile. At approximately this time the patient had succeeded in sitting up and in some walking with assistance. Therapy was shifted to another room where more objects of interest could be pointed out.

The nurse at this time commented on the patient's ability to sing simple songs with her as she was bathed and to count serially. While this latter was discouraged, since the writer had found previously that a continuous serial counting tended to slow the later use of numbers, the nurse apparently gained so much pleasure out of the counting during exercise and daily activity that it was continued. (The results of this behavior will be noted later. It should also be pointed out that the ability to sing simple songs in repetition does not point to successful verbalization and may retard free and voluntary speech.)

The nurse and family were encouraged to continue the naming process then being used in therapy. Writing as a substitute for speech was also encouraged, but at this time in therapy it lagged behind oral verbalization.

Physiotherapy, which had been a regular part of therapy, was continued on a three-times-a-week basis by a professional therapist. Walking with a cane and with the assistance of the nurse was also encouraged. Some success was obtained, and the patient slowly became ambulatory. Increased motivation for language was noted with the increased mobility. The patient was noted as being withdrawn and seclusive, however. Some of this attitude, it was felt, was due to the husband's emotional reaction to the patient's incapacity. Friends were discouraged from visiting the patient, although such socialization was urged by the therapist. (It was many months before the therapist could overcome this attitude in the husband and in the patient.) The patient's contacts were limited to the family, the nurse, the physiotherapist, the family physician, and the aphasia therapist. Because of the husband's rather extreme emotional reaction to the patient's abortive efforts to communicate, he played little part in the actual therapeusis at this time. A succession of nurses were hired and for one reason or another discharged. Most of them were incompetent as therapists or as assistants in the language instruction efforts. One nurse who stayed with the family for several months, however, proved to be stimulating and efficient. She accepted the role of language therapist and followed the process of therapy carefully and quite successfully. (Both of these problems, the emotionality of the family and the incompetence of household help, must be carefully evaluated before the people involved can be used in the therapeutic process. As noted, overemotionality on the part of the family will produce anxiety and emotional behavior in the patient which will negate therapy. Incompetence or failure to follow therapeutic suggestions by the nurse or other household help may actually retard therapy.)

As the word-naming process and beginning writing of word-names progressed, the therapy shifted to the second stage of language training. Verb forms were added. With each object named, the use of that object was demonstrated and the verb form given. For example, the word "book" evoked by pointing to a book was accompanied by the act of reading aloud from the book by the therapist. The word "read" was then spoken. The combination of "book read" was then used as the book was selected. As the daily paper was indicated and the word "paper" spoken by the patient, the same verb was added, making the combination "paper read." The same process was followed for magazines, theater programs, menus, and self-written sentences on paper until the act of reading was associated with the noun. Word combinations using the noun and verb forms were added in like manner for "pencil write," "water drink," etc. Later as the name-word was repeated or written, or the object was indicated by the therapist, the patient would add the use or verb form that accompanied it. In this way the two-word sentence was formed. Voluntary and free speech was still quite difficult, and language needed to be stimulated before it would be used by the patient. Many paraphasic errors were noted. The patient would reverse syllables, substitute sounds, elide endings, and telescope words. Attempted correction of these errors was noted as being quite futile. While the patient would sometimes correct the errors when they were pointed out, she often would be unable to correct them. It was noted that she rarely noted her own errors. (This failure at self-recognition of errors is common in the receptive aphasic patient.)

Beginning reading was attempted through single words found in newspaper headlines and in magazines. The reading was combined with writing and with oral attempts. For example, the word "book" was spoken as the object was indicated; the word was then written on a paper by the therapist and later by the patient; and the same word was searched for in the daily paper. As therapy continued, it was noted that reading could only be stimulated in this way. The patient read the daily paper assiduously but understood very little of what she read. The first direct attempts were limited to picture-reading and then to common words in headlines. (Size of print made a considerable difference here; some understanding was obtainable on very large words, but the same words in small print were quite difficult and frequently not comprehended.) The patient could not be motivated by books printed in large print for children. She was seen to react quite emotionally and even catastrophically when the attempt was made to introduce the books she herself had written. Consequently, reading was confined to word-selection from the newspapers, to flash-card words, and to words printed by the therapist. As time went on, smaller print was used and the patient was able to read the daily paper with some degree of comprehension. It was noted, however, that grammatical parts of speech such as prepositions, articles, interjections, and conjunctions were not understood. Silent reading progressed much more rapidly than oral reading.

At this time it was also noted that writing as a form of communication had advanced beyond the verbal form. Many words that the patient could not speak could be written. Spelling was difficult and at times made reading the written word extremely trying. Paraphasic errors were noted in the writing that paralleled the spoken form of paraphasia noted above. Errors of transposition, substitution, and elision were common. As in the spoken form, these errors were not self-corrected in most instances. The patient would recognize her inability to write a particular word to her satisfaction but would most often be unable to correct or complete words that were difficult for her. (This impotence is a consistent sign in brain-injured patients.)

At the patient's request, number work was started. It was at this point that the previous insistence of the nurse on serial counting was found to be a real deterrent to learning. So accommodated had the patient become to using numbers in a serial fashion that when she was shown a number, she could speak it only by counting up to it. This process so delayed the use of numbers that numerical problems were invariably confused and difficult. The patient did succeed in some addition of numbers but never got beyond that point. After a series of attempts which occupied part of each therapeutic session for several months, the patient lost all interest in using numbers or in working on the problems given to her. She succeeded in the practical use of numbers only for the days of the month and for telling time. This was almost invariably done by serialization. Making change was too difficult, since it meant counting backwards or subtraction, which the patient could not master. Prices of objects purchased could be understood but rarely repeated orally. Computation as a means of communication was never achieved.

As verbalization and language developed, it was noted that dysarthria and paraphasia played an increasing role. Speech which could be understood on the single-word level most of the time became quite unintelligible. Attempts were made through phonetics to reduce this phase of the problem. Success was obtained to some degree in the actual therapeutic sessions but was not seen to carry over to communication outside of the therapy. Socialization was urged continuously and to some degree achieved. The patient would go out for long rides each day. She was encouraged to talk whenever possible. Originally, this took the form of naming what she saw, later to naming and use, and still later to more complete sentence form. The latter was rarely achieved, however.

As the patient and her husband and the nurse went to various restaurants and the opportunity increased to see people daily who were familiar to her, some of the reserve with other people broke down. At the beginning she would indicate what she wanted to eat. At first this was a process of having the menu read to her and responding by nodding her head when something she wanted was mentioned. Later, she began to read the menu herself and then indicating it to the waitress. Later she attempted to read the menu aloud. Sometimes her attempts were understood, sometimes she could not be understood. At first this lack of understanding tended to make her withdraw, but later she became quite insistent and would repeat her demands until she was understood or the husband interpreted for the waitress. This outside behavior was carefully followed in therapy. Menu-reading and selection of a complete meal became a part of each session. During this period friends were encouraged to call. The patient's first reaction was to sit quietly and not attempt to enter into conversations. Later, she responded more and more with verbal and gestural language forms. These socializing efforts were also followed in therapy, and greetings and simple phrases that could be used were stressed. The patient evidenced a passing interest in moving pictures, but these needed to be at a high level, containing classical music presentation or classical plays. Most pictures were rejected. (This, it appeared, was the same pattern of picture-attendance that she had prior to her brain disorder.)

Her reading was limited to stories concerning social change or world politics. She became quite facile in reading long articles and abstracting the major meanings from them. For example, she once read a full column describing the war in the Middle East and when asked what the article was about she said "Oil and power." Her speech continued to be replete with dysarthric and paraphasic errors. It was felt that a change in environment might be beneficial and stimulating to her. The husband was encouraged to travel with her, and since the winter was becoming more severe, the family moved to California. This brought the direct therapy to an end.

Examination at the conclusion of direct therapy showed a residual mixed type of aphasia where both receptive and expressive features were present in almost every language sphere. The patient was noted as able to write, to read, and to speak with some degree of ease. Dysarthria and paraphasia were both seen to a fairly marked degree. The patient was more outgoing and could accept her handicap to some degree but was still easily frustrated and reacted emotionally to many language failures. From letters received from the patient it is evident that these problems still exist. She is ambulatory but remains unable to use her right arm. Hemiparesis still exists in the right leg. She is still euphoric at times but intermittently becomes depressed and anxious. She shows no basic change in her interests. Compared with her language ability at the beginning of therapy, she has shown considerable progress. This has not been sufficient to overcome the major part of her aphasic disturbance, however.

Conclusion

The two cases presented illustrate widely separate approaches to the problem of aphasia. They have been presented in some detail to show the behavior of the patients as well as to demonstrate the type of therapy which seemed indicated in the different apraxic and agnosic areas. The over-all approach where individual and group therapy can be used presents many instances of the value of controlled and guided therapeusis. It is believed to be an ideal therapeutic situation where all of the possible contributing therapies and therapists can be brought into the therapeusis. It is believed, however, that this can lead to very serious end-results unless the therapist is cautious. The in-patient situation easily becomes a dependency relationship. The patient becomes sheltered and overprotected from the external environment, which undoubtedly is threatening to him. During early stages of therapy this may be highly desirable, but, if it is continued too long, it becomes a very definite deterrent to rehabilitation. The goals of aphasia therapy must lie in the direction of establishing an independent attitude—an ability to relate to the environment of life at the patient's level—and not a false security of dependency. As was pointed out in the second case, the overprotective attitude of the husband of the patient led to a seclusiveness and a withdrawal from human contacts that needed to be dealt with continuously in therapy before the patient began to make definite outgoing efforts. It is believed that this to some degree delayed therapy.

The author believes that fundamentally aphasia therapy should not be conceived as a simple process of developing a new vocabulary or of adding newly learned language concepts. Rather, it must be a process of assisting the patient through a variety of stimulations in his groping toward ego-integrity through new cortical integrations by his remaining intact cortex. The patient must be motivated at succeeding levels and in many areas to attempt language based upon his previous learning, as encouraged through new stimuli. The therapist must be at various times a speech pathologist, a clinical psychologist, and an educator. He must possess infinite patience, considerable skill, and wide imagination. The problems posed by the aphasia patient require ingenuity and sufficient boldness to try new things as the situation requires. No absolute pathway to successful therapeusis for aphasia is available. Each patient presents his own façade of personality and language deficiencies. Each patient presents a great challenge equal to any in the wide category of problems believed amenable to therapy.

BIBLIOGRAPHY

1. Selected Reading References

ACKERLY, S. S., and BENTON, A. L. "Report of a Case of Bilateral Frontal Lobe Deficit." In *The Frontal Lobes,* Association for Research in Nervous and Mental Diseases, Vol. XXVII, chap. xxi, pp. 479–504. Baltimore: The Williams & Wilkins Co., 1948.

ANDERSON, J. O. "Aphasia from the Viewpoint of a Speech Pathologist," *Journal of Speech Disorders,* IX (September, 1934), 3–16.

ANDERSON, JEANNETTE. "*Is* Is Not the Verb for Aphasia," *Journal of Speech Disorders,* XI (June, 1946), 133–37.

BACKUS, OLLIS. "Rehabilitation of Aphasic Veterans," *Journal of Speech Disorders,* X (June, 1945), 153–61.

BASTIAN, H. D. *The Brain as an Organ of the Mind.* London: Kegan Paul, Trench, Trubner & Co., 1880.

——. *A Treatise on Aphasia.* London: H. K. Lewis, 1898.

BERRY, J. A. *Brain and Mind.* New York: The Macmillan Co., 1928.

BERRY, M. F., and EISENSON, J. *The Defective in Speech.* New York: Appleton-Century-Crofts, Inc., 1947.

BUCY, PAUL. "Organization of Central Nervous System Control of Muscular Activity," *Chicago Medical Society Bulletin,* April 30, 1949, pp. 836–66.

BUTFIELD, E., and ZANGWILL, O. "Re-education in Aphasia," *Journal of Neurology, Neurosurgery and Psychiatry,* IX (New Series), No. 2 (April, 1946), 75–79.

CHESHER, E. C. "Some Observations Concerning the Relation of Handedness to the Language Mechanism," *Bulletin of the Neurological Institute of New York,* IV (April, 1936), 556–62.

EISENSON, JON. "Aphasics: Observations and Tentative Conclusions," *Journal of Speech Disorders,* XII (September, 1947), 291–92.

FREEMAN, WALTER, and WATTS, JAMES W. *Psychosurgery.* Springfield, Ill.: Charles C. Thomas, Publisher, 1942.

FROESCHELS, E. *Speech Therapy.* Boston: Expression Co., 1933.

FROESCHELS, E., and JELLINEK, A. *Practice of Voice and Speech Therapy.* Boston: Expression Co., 1941.

FROESCHELS, E., et al. *Psychological Elements in Speech.* Boston: Expression Co., 1932.

GOLDSTEIN, KURT. *Aftereffects of Brain Injuries in War.* New York: Grune & Stratton, Inc., 1932.

——. *Language and Language Disturbances.* New York: Grune & Stratton, Inc., 1942.

——. "Mental Changes Due to Frontal Lobe Damage," *Journal of Psychology,* XVII (April, 1944), 185–97.

——. *The Organism.* New York: American Book Co., 1939.

GOLDSTEIN, MAX. *The Acoustic Method.* St. Louis: Laryngoscope Press, 1939.

GOWERS, W. R. *Diseases of the Brain.* London: J. & A. Churchill Ltd., 1885.

GRANICK, L. *Aphasia: A Guide to Retraining.* New York: Grune & Stratton, Inc., 1947.

HALSTEAD, WARD C. "Behavioral Effects of Lesions of the Frontal Lobe in Man," *Archives of Neurology and Psychiatry,* XL (October, 1939), 6–14.

——. *Brain and Intelligence.* Chicago: University of Chicago Press, 1948.

HALSTEAD, WARD C. "Preliminary Analysis of Grouping Behavior in Patients with Cerebral Injury," *Journal of Psychology,* XX (May, 1940), 6–14.

———. "Specialization of Behavioral Functions and the Frontal Lobes." In *The Frontal Lobes,* Association for Research in Nervous and Mental Diseases, Vol. XXVII, chap. ii, pp. 59–65. Baltimore: The Williams & Wilkins Co., 1948.

HALSTEAD, W. C., and WEPMAN, J. M. "The Halstead-Wepman Aphasia Screening Test," *Journal of Speech and Hearing Disorders,* XIV (March, 1949), 9–15.

———. *Manual for the Halstead-Wepman Aphasia Screening Test.* Chicago: Departments of Medicine, Surgery, and Psychology, University of Chicago, 1949.

HARROWER-ERICKSON, M. R. "Personality Changes Accompanying Cerebral Lesions," *Archives of Neurology and Psychiatry,* XLIII (1940), 859–90.

HEAD, HENRY. *Aphasia and Kindred Disorders of Speech.* 2 vols. New York: The Macmillan Co., 1926.

HEBB, D. O. "Man's Frontal Lobes," *Archives of Neurology and Psychiatry,* LIV (July, 1945), 10–24.

JACKSON, HUGHLINGS. "Selected Writings of J. Hughlings Jackson," edited by Henry Head, *Brain,* XXXVIII (October, 1915), 1–90.

KENNEDY, F., and WOLF, A. "The Relation of Intellect to Speech Defect in Aphasia Patients," *Journal of Nervous and Mental Diseases,* LXXXIV (August, 1936), 125–26.

KUPPER, H. I. "Psychic Concomitants in Wartime Injuries," *Psychomatic Medicine,* VII (January, 1945), 15–21.

LASHLEY, K. S. "Factors Limiting Recovery After Central Nervous System Lesions," *Journal of Nervous and Mental Diseases,* LXXXVIII (October, 1938), 733–55.

———. "Functional Determinants of Cerebral Localization," *Archives of Neurology and Psychiatry,* XXXVIII (August, 1937), 371–87.

LINN, L., and STEIN, M. H. "Sodium Amytal in Treatment of Aphasia," *Bulletin of the U. S. Army Medical Department,* V (June, 1946), 705–8.

MALMO, R. H. "Psychological Aspects of Frontal Gyrectomy and Frontal Lobotomy in Mental Patients." In *The Frontal Lobes,* Association for Research in Nervous and Mental Diseases, Vol. XXVII, chap. xxiii, Part 3, pp. 537–64. Baltimore: The Williams & Wilkins Co., 1948.

MILLS, CHARLES. "Aphasia and the Cerebral Zones of Speech," *American Journal of Medical Science,* XVI (March, 1904), 375–93.

———. "The Naming Center," *Journal of Nervous and Mental Diseases,* XXI (January, 1895), 1016–22.

———. "Treatment of Aphasia by Training," *Journal of the American Medical Association,* XLIII (May, 1904), 1940–49.

NIELSEN, J. M. *Agnosia, Apraxia, Aphasia.* New York: Paul B. Hoeber, Inc., Medical Book Department of Harper & Bros., 1946.

———. "The Cortical Motor Pattern Apraxias." In *The Frontal Lobes,* Association for Research in Nervous and Mental Diseases, Vol. XXVII, chap. xxiv, pp. 565–81. Baltimore: The Williams & Wilkins Co., 1948.

PEACHER, W. G. "Speech Disorders in World War II," *Journal of Speech Disorders,* X (June, 1945), 155–58.

PENFIELD, W., and EVANS, J. "The Frontal Lobe in Man," *Brain,* LVIII (April, 1935), 115–33.

PENFIELD, W., and ERICKSON, T. C. *Epilepsy and Cerebral Localization.* Springfield, Ill.: Charles C. Thomas, Publisher, 1941.

PENFIELD, W., and RASMUSSEN, T. *The Cerebral Cortex of Man.* New York: The Macmillan Co., 1950.

PIERON, HENRI. *Thought and Brain.* London: Kegan Paul, Trench, Trubner & Co., 1927.

SALL, M., and WEPMAN, J. M. "A Screening Survey of Organic Impairment," *Journal of Speech Disorders,* X (May, 1945), 283–86.

SHEEHAN, VIVIAN. "Rehabilitation of Aphasias in an Army Hospital," *Journal of Speech Disorders,* XI (June, 1946), 152–59.
University of Michigan Speech Clinic Staff. *Aphasia in Adults.* Ann Arbor, Mich.: University of Michigan Press, 1947.
VAN RIPER, C. *Speech Correction.* New York: Prentice-Hall, Inc., 1947.
WECHSLER, ISRAEL. *Textbook of Clinical Neurology.* Philadelphia: W. B. Saunders Co., 1939.
WEPMAN, JOSEPH M. "Organization of Aphasia Therapy," *Journal of Speech Disorders,* XII (December, 1947), 405–9.
WEST, R., KENNEDY, L., and CARR, A. *Rehabilitation of Speech.* Rev. ed.; New York: Harper & Bros., 1947.
WEISENBURG, T., and McBRIDE, K. *Aphasia.* New York: The Commonwealth Fund, Division of Publications, 1935.
ZOLLINGER, R. "Removal of Left Cerebral Hemisphere," *Archives of Neurology and Psychiatry,* XXXIV (November, 1935), 1055–64.

2. Selected Practice Materials

DOLCH, E. W. *A Manual for Remedial Reading.* Champaign, Ill.: The Garrard Press, 1945.
FERNALD, G. M. *Remedial Techniques in Basic School Subjects.* New York: McGraw-Hill Book Co., Inc., 1943.
FREEMAN, F. N. *Correlated Handwriting: Practice Books 1, 2, and 3.* Columbus, O.: Zaner-Bloser Co., 1931.
GARDNER, WARREN. *Left-handed Writing.* Danville, Ill.: Interstate Press, 1945.
GATES, ARTHUR. *Improvement in Reading.* New York: The Macmillan Co., 1947.
GRAY, WILLIAM S. *On Their Own in Reading.* Chicago: Scott, Foresman & Co., 1948.
GRISWOLD, L. *Handicraft.* Colorado Springs, Colo.: Outwest Printing and Stationery Co., 1945.
HILGARD, E. R. *Theories of Learning.* New York: Appleton-Century-Crofts, Inc., 1948.
ICKIS, M. *Pastimes for the Patient.* New York: A. S. Barnes & Co., Inc., 1945.
New Trend Arithmetic-Skill Texts, Books 2–8. Columbus, O.: Charles E. Merrill Co., 1945.
PRESCOTT, D. E. *Emotions and the Educative Process.* Washington, D. C.: American Council on Education, 1938.
STIERI, E. *The Book of Indoor Living.* New York: Whittlesey House, 1946.
TROWBRIDGE, C. R. *Feeling Better?* New York: Dodd, Mead & Co., Inc., 1936.

INDEX OF NAMES

INDEX OF SUBJECTS

Calculation apraxia, 132 f., 229, 251
  serial counting in, 261
  therapy for, 229 f.
Case histories, 250–56, 257–62
Case histories, extracts of, 133, 137, 172, 174 f.
Central aphasia, 38
Climate, 91 f., 117, 128
Clinics, university, 5, 112, 116
Conduction aphasia, 38
Construction apraxia, 132 f., 230, 251
  therapy for, 230 f.
Contralateral cortical control, 27
Convolution,
  first temporal, 10
  third frontal, 9 f., 14
Cortical aphasia, 38
Cortical integration, 263
  total, 15
Cortical sensory aphasia, 38
Counseling, 3

Diaschisis (von Monakow), 22
Diet, 168 f.
Disintegration, Goldstein's laws of, 17
Dominant hemisphere, 12, 81
Dysarthria, 30 f., 105, 112, 120, 132 f., 150, 213, 240, 251, 262
  therapy for, 111, 240 f.
Dysdiadokokinesia, 112
Dysphasia, 65

Educational history, 121
Electroencephalography, 31, 120
Epilepsy; see Seizures
Etiology of aphasia
  aneurysm, 133
  brain tumor, 30, 50, 116
  brain-tumor extirpation, 5
  cerebral accidents, 174
  cerebral thrombosis, 30
  cerebro-vascular accidents, 257
  cerebro-vascular disease, 50
  head injury, 5, 50
  trauma, direct, 172
Expressive aphasia, 37, 41, 50 ff., 54, 58, 61, 63 f., 69, 73, 76 f., 86, 172, 213, 234, 251
  Broca's aphasia, 9
  predominant expressive difficulty, 37
  self-criticism in, 172
  therapy for, 234 ff.
Expressive-impressive aphasia, 37
Expressive-receptive aphasia, 37, 42, 50 ff., 54, 58, 61, 63 f., 69, 73, 76 f., 86, 111, 119, 133, 244, 257
  therapy for, 245 f.

Family,
  effect of, on patients, 259
  emotional reaction of, to patients, 259
  interviews with, 126
  relationships, 123
Fingeragnosie (Gerstmann), 39, 208
Frontal gyrus, third left, 29
Frontal lobe,
  activity controlled by, 17, 20
  and bilateral lobotomies, 25
  and bilateral gyrectomies, 25
  and catastrophic reactions, 23
  and concrete behavior, 25
  discussion of, 17, 22 f.
  and expressive signs, 119
  and frontal lobectomies, 21, 23
  Halstead's four-factor theory and, 88

General (nonverbal) apraxia, 132 f., 213 f., 251
  therapy for, 214 ff.
Gestalt, 16, 80 f., 113, 159
Gestural language, 262
Ghost-of-the-past, 173
Global aphasia, 42, 50 ff., 58, 61, 63 f., 69, 73, 76 f., 86, 111, 244
  therapy for, 245 ff.

Halstead's four-factor theory, 21 f., 88, 119
  abstraction factor, 21
  central integrative field factor, 21, 113
  directional factor, 22
  power factor, 21, 33, 88, 113, 119

Ideokinetic apraxia, 132 f., 232, 251
  therapy for, 232 ff.
Impressive aphasia, 37
Initial aphasia, 50
Instructors, use of, 56
Integrative function of the cortex, 110, 162
Intelligence, 70–75, 77 ff.
  biological, 164, 169
  changes in, 75
  defects of, 70 f.
  deterioration in, 48, 125
  disorganization of, 25
  generalized loss of, 171
  impairment of, 33, 129
  judgment of, 147 f.
  measurement of, 48, 71 ff., 127
  and memory, 148 f.
  nonverbal, 48
Introspective reports by patients, 92–96
Irreminiscence (Nielsen), 39

Jargon aphasia, 30, 39

Left brain, doctrine of, 28 ff., 81
Left-handedness, 28, 30